Strategies for the Future of Nursing

Strategies for the Future of Nursing

Changing Roles, Responsibilities, and Employment Patterns of Registered Nurses

Edward O'Neil

Janet Coffman

Editors

Sponsored by
The Center for the Health Professions
at the University of California,
San Francisco

Jossey-Bass Publishers
San Francisco

Substantial discounts on bulk quantities of Jossey-Bass books
are available to corporations, professional associations, and
other organizations. For details and discount information, contact the special sales department at Jossey-Bass Inc., Publishers
(415) 433–1740; Fax (800) 605–2665.

For sales outside the United States, please contact your
local Simon & Schuster International Office.
www.josseybass.com

TCF   Manufactured in the United States of America on Lyons
Falls Turin Book. This paper is acid-free and 100 percent totally
chlorine-free.

Library of Congress Cataloging-in-Publication Data

Strategies for the future of nursing : changing roles,
responsibilities, and employment patterns of registered nurses /
Edward O'Neil, Janet Coffman, editors. — 1st ed.
p.   cm.
Contents: the changing health care environment / Edward O'Neil—
Trends in the nursing workforce and nursing education / Janet
Coffman, Noelle Blick, and Sabrina Wong—Projecting the future
supply and demand for registered nurses / Edward Salsberg,
Paul Wing, and Carol S. Brewer—The impact of managed care and
integrated delivery systems on demand for registered nurses /
Barbara Balik—The changing demand for registered nurses in
hospitals / Maryann F. Fralic—Registered nurses in long-term care /
Charlene Harrington—Opportunities and challenges for registered
nurses in ambulatory care and community-based settings / Janis P.
Bellack—Community-based nursing : exploring new frontiers while
reclaiming old territory / Marjorie K. Bauman—The changing role of
the advanced practice nurse / Catherine L. Gilliss and Mary O.
Mundinger—From case to medical care management : implications for
nursing education / Barry R. Greene and Debra L. Kelsey—Nursing
in the next century / Edward O'Neil.
ISBN 0-7879-4028-3 (cloth : acid-free paper)
1. Nursing—Practice—United States.   2. Nursing—United States—
Forecasting.   I. O'Neil, Edward H.   II. Coffman, Janet, [date].

RT86.73.S87   1998
610.73'01'12—dc21   97-45454
                                                               CIP

                           FIRST EDITION
HC Printing   10 9 8 7 6 5 4 3 2 1

CONTENTS

LIST OF TABLES AND FIGURES

Tables

Figures

PREFACE

This is a dislocating and, at times, frightening period for all health care professionals. The once stable environment of health care and professional practice is now marked by new relationships, shifting alliances, disappearing funding, and a set of expectations that is as changeable as it is novel. In such a world it is important to be able to assess where reality is and where it is likely to be headed. How do the challenges today relate to where institutions and professionals have been and where they are headed? The purpose of this book is to provide the nursing professional with just such an orientation.

The book is intended for every nurse in a leadership position, from hospitals and health care systems to education and managed care companies. It addresses issues ranging from the concerns of leading small groups of nurses in clinical settings to how nurses are positioned for the emerging megahealth care systems. The authors of each chapter have explored the unique opportunities that exist for the nursing profession in this emergent system. As well, they suggest the best strategies to securing these opportunities for the profession.

In the first chapter Edward O'Neil sets the stage by presenting a broad overview of recent changes in health care delivery and financing in the United States, which draws upon the author's ongoing work on this topic. The chapter points to those developments in the health care revolution that are particularly susceptible to a new role for nursing. O'Neil is associate professor of family and community medicine and codirector of the Center for the Health Professions at the University of California, San Francisco, and executive director of the Pew Health Professions Commission.

Janet Coffman, Noelle Blick, and Sabrina Wong, of the Center for the Health Professions at UCSF, provide an overview of trends in the nursing workforce and nursing education in Chapter Two. They address questions such as, What are the characteristics of the registered nurse (RN) workforce, and how has it changed over the past twenty years? What are the parallel trends in nursing education? This chapter is intended to provide background information about these trends, which are explored in greater depth in other chapters.

Edward Salsberg, Paul Wing, and Carol S. Brewer discuss the changing demand for and supply of RNs in the health care workforce in the third chapter. Faced with increased pressure to provide quality care at the lowest possible cost, health care delivery organizations are scrutinizing costs more closely than ever before. Given that RNs are the largest health care occupation and that labor constitutes the highest variable cost in health care, many cost containment efforts focus on RN staffing. These developments raise many questions about future demand for RNs. Estimates vary widely, with some experts projecting a steady increase in demand and others large job losses in the hospital sector. This chapter seeks to make sense of these conflicting projections by examining differences in forecasters' assumptions that influence their projections. The authors consider both aggregate demand for RNs and demand for RNs by educational level, identifying a deficit in the number of RNs educated at the bachelor's level and above. They offer policy recommendations to bring the mix of RNs by educational level in line with demand.

Barbara Balik of Allina Health Systems surveys the impact of the growth of managed care and *integrated delivery systems* on the roles, responsibilities, and employment patterns of RNs. Written with the insights gained from one of the nation's preeminent integrated delivery systems, Chapter Four begins by tracing health care market evolution, identifying the major activities occurring at each stage. The chapter then describes the roles and responsibilities of RNs in mature integrated delivery systems, using examples from Allina as illustrations. The author describes Allina's competency-based approach to RN staffing and the consequences of this approach for RN education.

New roles for nurses are emerging in a variety of new systems, simultaneously with dramatic changes in their roles in the *traditional hospital setting*. Hospitals continue to employ more RNs than any other health care sector. Written by Maryann F. Fralic, the chief nursing executive of the Johns Hopkins University Hospital, Chapter Five describes the evolution of hospitals' role in health care delivery and its consequences for their utilization of RNs. The chapter identifies increased acuity and pace of hospital care as factors precipitating an increase in the number of bachelor's prepared RNs demanded by hospitals.

Charlene Harrington, a national expert on the nursing home industry, provides critical insight into the changing RN role in long-term care in Chapter Six. It details the evolution of this industry and the roles of RNs in delivering care to nursing home residents. The author emphasizes the major role of public policy in shaping demand for RNs in nursing homes, which are reimbursed primarily by the Medicare and Medicaid programs. She argues persuasively that political constraints on public spending for health care services for the elderly and disabled are likely to restrict growth in RN employment in nursing homes. In addition, the author discusses inadequate educational preparation as a potential risk to quality nursing home care. However, as with ambulatory care, a shift to long-term care settings probably will not result in a shift in RN job opportunities of equal magnitude.

The ambulation of care out of the hospital and into the community has been a sustained trend for over a decade. Janis P. Bellack, from the Medical University of South Carolina, looks to how technological advances, coupled with pressures to contain costs and prevent illness, have led to a *rapid expansion of the delivery of health care services in ambulatory settings.* Chapter Seven describes the various ambulatory settings in which RNs are employed and their roles and responsibilities in these settings. The author highlights major differences between the RN staffing patterns of hospitals and ambulatory care providers, the latter of which typically use fewer RNs and more advanced practice nurses than hospitals.

As care moves out of hospitals, community-based RN services are enjoying a renaissance of sorts as the population ages and health care delivery systems strive to minimize hospital utilization. Marjorie K. Bauman, the executive in charge of the Johns Hopkins Home Care Group, looks at the growth of home health agencies and the new opportunities they offer RNs in Chapter Eight. This chapter traces the evolution of community-based RN services from the public health nurses of the turn of the century to today's home health RNs. The author describes the impact of Medicare as well as other market forces on the ever-changing roles and responsibilities of RNs in home care. The current environment suggests an increased demand for RNs with strong independent judgment and critical thinking skills typically acquired at the bachelor's level as well as for RNs with master's level training in administration and specialized clinical fields.

This volume also addresses the enormous opportunities that the changing system is presenting to the advanced practice nurse (APN) in all practice settings. APNs are the fastest-growing segment of the RN workforce. Written by Catherine L. Gilliss and Mary O'Neil Mundinger, two of the nation's leaders in APN education, Chapter Nine describes the various factors shaping demand for APNs in both ambulatory and hospital settings. The authors discuss the potential dampening effects on demand for APNs due to the oversupply of physicians and the concomitant shift in new physicians' interests from specialist to generalist careers. The authors also assess similarities and differences between APN and physician assistant education.

Barry R. Greene and Debra L. Kelsey offer a perspective from managed care as to how the nurse might play an expanded role in population-based care systems. Chapter Ten focuses on the growing utilization of RNs to manage the health of both individuals and populations. The chapter begins by describing the development of medical management as a strategy for managing the delivery of a full spectrum of services to a population and the emerging roles and responsibilities of RNs in providing medical management services. The authors detail the knowledge and skills required of RNs in medical management roles, highlighting the gap between employers' needs and RNs' educational preparation. The final section of the chapter outlines a framework for revamping RN education to ensure that RNs have the critical thinking and applied research skills necessary to function effectively as medical care managers.

What do these changes in RNs' roles, responsibilities, and employment patterns portend for RN education and practice? Edward O'Neil concludes the book with seven recommended strategic actions for nurses, nursing education, and nursing professional organizations. These actions are critical to securing the opportunities that are reviewed throughout the book.

February 1998
San Francisco

Edward O'Neil
Janet Coffman

ACKNOWLEDGMENTS

We have incurred great debts to numerous colleagues and friends over the course of this project.

Greatest thanks are due the authors who contributed chapters to this book. We thank them not only for their talent and dedication but also for their patience and understanding. All are professionals in every sense of the word.

The advisory committee for this project deserves much credit for shaping this book's focus and scope. Colleen Conway-Welch, Rheba de Tornyay, Maryann F. Fralic, and Barry R. Greene provided strong leadership and support at every stage of the project.

The chapters of this book are derived from papers presented at a symposium held in San Francisco, California, in June 1996. We thank James Blumstein, Peter Buerhaus, Theresa Cosca, Dorothy Deremo, Mary Lou Hennrich, David Reynolds, Thomas Rundall, and Edward Salsberg for their thoughtful formal commentaries on individual papers. Colleen Conway-Welch, Rheba de Tornyay, Barbara Donaho, and Marla Salmon rose to the formidable challenge of summarizing the papers' findings and their implications. Arlyss Anderson-Rothman, Carolyn Asbury, Marilyn Chow, Julie Morath, Jane Norbeck, Barbara Norrish, and Joanne Spetz also participated in the symposium, offering many thoughtful insights.

A number of individuals provided invaluable assistance with the editing of the manuscript. Stephanie Bobo contributed expert copyediting essential to converting the papers into book chapters. Arnold Kaluzny reviewed the entire manuscript, offering important suggestions for improving its organization and internal coherence. An expanded advisory committee carefully reviewed the closing chapter. Carolyn Asbury, Barbara Balik, Colleen Conway-Welch, Rheba de Tornyay, Barbara Donaho, Maryann F. Fralic, Barry R. Greene, Sherrie Hans, Debra L. Kelsey, and Marla Salmon offered critical insights, many of which were incorporated into the final draft of this chapter.

We are most grateful to the staff of Jossey-Bass, Inc., for their patience and expertise. Andrew Pasternack, editor of Jossey Bass's Health Series, quickly recognized the project's importance and patiently nudged us along to completion. Adrienne Chieng provided thorough assistance with editorial details. Madhu Prasher, Frank Welsch, and Marcella Friel shepherded the manuscript through the production phase. Margaret Seabold and her staff coordinated communications. Jennifer Morley and Jennifer Zahgkuni served as our liaisons with the marketing department.

This project would not have been possible without the generous financial support of the Pew Charitable Trusts. Carolyn Asbury, former director of health and human services, assisted greatly in the development and implementation of this project. Sherrie Hans, program officer in the health and human services division, participated in later stages of the project, providing a fresh perspective on our efforts.

Words cannot adequately express the debt we owe our colleagues at the UCSF Center for the Health Professions. Several individuals made special contributions to our work. When not sharing their wit, wisdom, and steadfast moral support, Catherine L. Gilliss and Janis P. Bellack found time to author chapters. Sabrina Wong brought great energy, enthusiasm, and dedication to several stages of the project. Her assistance was essential to the success of the symposium and production of the final manuscript. Noelle Blick also coauthored a chapter and assisted in the editing of several papers. Beth Mertz gave keen attention to the details of checking references and updating data. Ann Clarke oversaw our budget and preparations for the symposium. Meghan O'Keefe and Jonathan King provided critical administrative support.

Finally, we are grateful to our friends and families, who have had to live with us as we struggled to transform our ideas into a finished product. Thank you for the love, loyalty, support, and companionship without which this book would not have been possible.

E.O.
J.C.

THE EDITORS

Edward O'Neil is an associate professor of family and community medicine at the University of California, San Francisco, where he also serves as codirector of the Center for the Health Professions. Since 1989, O'Neil has also served as the executive director of the Pew Health Professions Commission.

Prior to taking his position at UCSF, O'Neil was assistant dean of medical education at Duke University, where he was also associate professor in the Department of Public Policy. He has also served as codirector of both the Pew Veterinary Medical and Dental Education Programs. In addition, he was associate dean at the School of Dentistry at the University of North Carolina at Chapel Hill and a program associate with the W. K. Kellogg Foundation.

O'Neil serves on the board of numerous organizations, including the School of Public Health at the University of California, Berkeley, the California Health Care Collaborative, the American Academy of Pediatric Dentistry Foundation, and the National Fund for Medical Education, for which he is vice chairman of the board and chairman of the executive committee.

O'Neil's numerous awards and honors include outstanding service recognition from the American Association of Dental Schools and membership in Omicron Delta Upsilon, Dental Honorary Fraternity.

Janet Coffman is associate director for workforce policy and analysis at the UCSF Center for the Health Professions. She received a master's degree in public policy from the University of California, Berkeley, in 1995. Prior to attending UC-Berkeley, she served on the staff of the U.S. Senate Committee on Veterans' Affairs, participating in the development of major legislation concerning salaries for VA's registered nurses, physicians, and dentists. Coffman also holds bachelor's and master's degrees in history from Haverford College (1988) and the State University of New York at Binghamton (1989), respectively.

Coffman's work at the center focuses on analysis of supply and demand for health professionals and development of recommendations for reform of health professions education policy. Coffman serves on the advisory committee for the California Strategic Planning Committee for Nursing: Colleagues in Caring for Nursing, a nursing workforce initiative funded by the Robert Wood Johnson Foundation.

Coffman is coauthor of "Physicians and Nurse Practitioners—Old Conflicts and New Opportunities," published in the *Western Journal of Medicine* in 1996.

THE CONTRIBUTORS

Barbara Balik is the patient care vice president at United Hospital, a major facility within the Allina Health System of St. Paul, Minnesota. She received her B.S.N. from Marycrest College and her MS in maternal-child health nursing from the University of Minnesota, and is currently a doctoral student at the University of St. Thomas. She has facilitated major redesign and other activities to ensure cross-functional team development in managed care environments.

Her main research activities have focused on health care organizational change, patient care practices, and children's health. She contributed the chapters "Partnership in Care" in *Patient as Partner* (1997) and "The Human Side of Change—Transition to Teams" in *Nurses as Patient Care Administrators: Strategic Perspective and Application* (1998).

Balik has served as president and board member of the Twin Cities Organization of Nurse Executives. She is a Wharton Fellow and received the Sigma Theta Tau, Zeta Chapter Leadership Award and the Minnesota Nurses Association Service Award.

Marjorie K. Bauman is currently president and chief executive officer of Johns Hopkins Home Care Group, Inc., Baltimore, Maryland. Having received her BSN (1969) from St. Olaf College in Minnesota and her MS (1973) from the University of Colorado, Bauman has dedicated twenty-five years of her career to public health and home health care clinical practice, advanced practice, education of nursing students at the baccalaureate level, home care research, and public health and home health administration. Her accomplishments include founding two home health agencies and managing a national study of outcomes-based quality measures for home health care.

Bauman's main research activities have focused on the development of outcome measures for Medicare home health. She has published articles on outcome measurement and quality improvement approaches in community-based nursing practice.

Bauman is a member of the Board of Priority Partners, a managed care organization. She has also had experience as a Joint Commission on the Accreditation of Healthcare Organizations surveyor of home health agencies. Her awards include Sigma Theta Tau, Who's Who in American Nursing, and Who's Who Among Top Executives.

Janis P. Bellack is currently associate provost for education and professor of nursing and health professions at the Medical University of South Carolina. She also holds a joint appointment as director of nursing programs for the statewide South Carolina Area Health Education Consortium. Bellack is also a senior fellow at the Center for the Health Professions at the University of California, San Francisco.

A graduate of the last diploma nursing class at the University of Virginia, Bellack subsequently earned her BSN (1970) at the same institution. She also holds a MN (1971) in pediatric nursing from the University of Florida, and a PhD (1987) in educational policy studies and evaluation from the University of Kentucky. Previously, Bellack held faculty positions at the University of Virginia, Old Dominion University, and the University of Kentucky.

Bellack is a fellow of the American Academy of Nursing and a member of Sigma Theta Tau International. She is the current president of the South Carolina League for Nursing and a member of the executive committee of the NLN Council on Baccalaureate and Higher Degree Programs.

Bellack's research focuses on health professions education. She has published numerous articles on nursing education and practice, as well as a nursing textbook, *Nursing Assessment and Diagnosis: A Multidimensional Approach* (2nd ed., 1992). She also serves on the editorial boards of the *On-Line Journal of Nursing Issues* and the *Journal of Nursing Education*.

Noelle Blick spent eight years in clinical work as a paramedic before entering college to pursue a degree in public health. She graduated from San Francisco State University with a bachelor of arts in health sciences in 1996. Blick has worked in a variety of clinical, administrative, research, and policy positions concerning issues of emergency medical response, AIDS, HIV-positive youth, and homelessness. She is currently working at the UCSF Center for the Health Professions on issues relating to state regulation of health professionals.

Carol S. Brewer is an assistant professor of nursing at the State University of New York at Buffalo. She earned her BSN degree (1977) from Trenton State College. She earned her MSN (1983) from the University of Tennessee, Knoxville, and both an MA in applied economics (1991) and a Ph.D. in nursing (1994, in administration and health care systems) from the University of Michigan.

Brewer's research focus has been on the nursing labor workforce. She has presented and published on the nursing labor supply, labor models, and other issues in nursing workforce research. Brewer has worked extensively with data from the National Sample Surveys of Registered Nurses, and has also conducted research on nurse staffing issues and workforce in western New York.

Brewer is a member of Phi Beta Kappa and Sigma Theta Tau. She currently serves on the board of the New York State Organization of Nurse Executives.

Maryann F. Fralic is vice president for nursing at The Johns Hopkins Hospital and associate dean of The Johns Hopkins University School of Nursing. Fralic formerly served as senior vice president of nursing at Robert Wood Johnson University Hospital in New Brunswick, New Jersey, and as clinical associate dean at Rutgers University College of Nursing. She holds a doctorate in health services administration from the University of Pittsburgh, where she was assistant professor of nursing administration.

Fralic is chairman of the National Advisory Committee for the Ladders in Nursing Careers project, a Robert Wood Johnson Foundation initiative for minority and economically disadvantaged health care workers. She serves on the National Advisory Council on Nurse Education and Practice and has served on many other advisory bodies, including the Pew Health Professions Commission's Advisory Panel on Nursing. Fralic was also a member of the Nursing Standards Task Force that developed the Joint Commission on Accreditation of Healthcare Organizations' current nursing standards.

Fralic's many honors include election to the American Academy of Nursing and the National Academies of Practice. She is also a fellow in the Johnson & Johnson-Wharton Program in Management for Nurses. In addition, Fralic serves on the editorial boards of the *Journal of Nursing Administration, Nursing Leadership Forum,* and *Nursing Connections.*

Catherine L. Gilliss is professor and chair of the Department of Family Health Care Nursing at the University of California, San Francisco. She is also a senior fellow at the UCSF Center for the Health Professions. A BSN graduate of Duke University (1971), she also holds a MSN (1974) from Catholic University of America and a DNSc (1983) from UCSF. Gilliss has held nursing faculty positions at the University of Maryland, Catholic University of America, University of Portland, and Sonoma State University.

She is the immediate past president of the National Organization of Nurse Practitioner Faculties and a winner of its Outstanding Nurse Practitioner Educator award. Gilliss completed a USPHS Primary Care Policy Fellowship in 1993 and is a Robert Wood Johnson Fellow in primary care. She is a fellow of the American Academy of Nursing.

Gilliss's scientific interests include the family and chronic illness and primary care workforce issues. She has written numerous articles and book chapters and edited several books. Her most recent chapter, coauthored by L. Davis, is "Primary Care for the 21st Century: The Future for Advanced Practice Nurses" in *Joining Forces: Articulating the Advanced Practice Role of Professional Nursing* (M. McCarthy and C. Sheehy, editors; 1998).

Gilliss chairs the Nursing Science Review Committee, Study Section (National Institute for Nursing Research).

Barry R. Greene is vice president of research of the Center for Research in Ambulatory Health Care Administration, the research arm of Medical Group Management Association.

Greene's thirty-year career has been dominated by health care administration research and teaching. He previously served as professor and chair of the University of Florida's Department of Health Services Administration and director of its graduate program. Greene also served as an associate dean in the University of Florida's College of Health Related Professions. Prior to that, he was a faculty member at Yale University, the University of Minnesota, and Trinity University.

Greene has also served as chair of the Accrediting Commission on Education for Health Services Administration and the Association of University Programs in Health Administration. He was also a member of the Pew Health Professions Commission Advisory Panel.

Green has published many journal articles and contributed a chapter to the forthcoming book *Ambulatory Care Management* (3rd ed., edited by Ross and Williams). He also has been the principal investigator of numerous grant-funded health care services research projects.

Among his many honors, Greene was awarded successive fellowships from the Kellogg Foundation from 1973 to 1975 for responsibilities as a staff associate to the Accrediting Commission on Graduate Education for Health Services Administration. He also earned the HIAA/AUPHA Fellowship.

Greene earned his doctorate in sociology/health services research at St. Louis University in 1971, his master's in psychology at Northern Illinois University in DeKalb, and his bachelor's in psychology at Wartburg College at Waverly, Iowa. He did postdoctoral work at Yale University Medical School in 1976–77.

Charlene Harrington has a PhD in sociology and higher education from the University of California, Berkeley. She is professor and immediate past chair of the

Department of Social and Behavioral Sciences, School of Nursing, University of California, San Francisco. She is a fellow of the American Academy of Nursing and a member of the Institute of Medicine.

Harrington has had a long-standing interest in nursing home issues that began when she was director of the California State Licensing and Certification program, responsible for nursing home, hospital, and home health care regulation. She served on the Institute of Medicine's Committee to Study Nursing Home Regulation (1985–86) and the Institute of Medicine Committee on Nurse Staffing in Hospitals and Nursing Homes (1995–96).

In her seventeen years of research experience at UCSF, she has completed numerous research studies and articles on nursing home quality, supply, access, and consumer information. She has been the principal investigator for several large national research studies on state policies concerning long-term care funded by the Health Care Financing Administration and the Agency for Health Care Policy and Research. She recently coedited (with Carol Estes) a 1997 second edition of *Health Policy and Nursing*.

Debra L. Kelsey is an independent health care consultant with over eighteen years of clinical and operations experience. In her current role as a consultant, she provides services on managed care and medical management to health plans, management service organizations, and providers. She specializes in the areas of clinical integration, integrated delivery systems, quality standards, and managed care information systems. She earned her BS degree (1986) in health arts and her MHSA degree (1995) at the College of St. Francis, graduating from both programs with academic distinction.

Kelsey recently served as director of medical management at the University of Ilinois at Chicago's UIHMO, Inc., where she was responsible for the development, implementation, and oversight of a full-risk, delegated medical management program for the university's Medicaid HMO product. Before joining UIHMO, she was a senior consultant at the Blue Cross and Blue Shield Association in Chicago for four years.

Kelsey's grounding in clinical issues is based upon seven years of acute and ambulatory care nursing experience, as well as more broad-based experiences in developing disease management, outcomes measurement, and clinical guidelines-based programs.

Mary O'Neil Mundinger is the Centennial Professor in health policy and dean of the Columbia University School of Nursing. She has also held the positions of director of graduate programs at Columbia University and assistant professor at Pace University School of Nursing.

In 1996 she was elected president of Friends of the National Institute for Nursing Research. She is a fellow of the Institute of Medicine, the Association of Academic Health Policy, the National Academy of Practice, and the American Academy of Nursing. In 1993 she was appointed by President Clinton to the Health Professions Review Group. In 1984–85 she received a Robert Wood Johnson Health Policy Fellowship and from 1990 to 1993 served on the program's board.

Mundinger received her BSN degree from the University of Michigan and her MA degree from Columbia University Teachers College. She holds a doctorate in public health from Columbia. In 1996 she was awarded an honorary doctorate from Hamilton College. She is primarily known for her work on the impact of federal policy on community-based health care and home care issues for children, the elderly, and disadvantaged families. She is the author of *Home Care Controversy: Too Little, Too Late, Too Costly* (1983) and *Autonomy in Nursing* (1980).

Edward Salsberg is director of the Center for Health Workforce Studies and clinical associate professor at the School of Public Health, at the State University of New York at Albany. The center collects, analyzes, and disseminates data and information on the supply, demand, distribution, and use of health workers. Prior to establishing the Center for Health Workforce Studies, Salsberg was director of the Bureau of Health Resources Development for the New York State Department of Health for twelve years.

Salsberg is a senior fellow of the Center for the Health Professions and a member of the steering committee for the National Academy for State Health Policy. He has written numerous reports and is a frequent speaker on issues related to the health professions. Salsberg coauthored the *State Health Personnel Handbook* (with Paul Wing, 1995) and *Data Systems to Support State Health Personnel Planning and Policy Making* (with Paul Wing, 1992). He is also author of *State Strategies for Financing Graduate Medical Education* (1997).

Salsberg holds a master's degree in public administration from New York University's Wagner School (1974). In 1995 Salsberg received the Second Century Award from the Columbia University School of Nursing.

Paul Wing is deputy director of the Center for Health Workforce Studies at the School of Public Health at the University at Albany. Wing earned his BS degree (1962) in basic engineering from Princeton University, and both his MA degree (1968) in statistics and his doctor of engineering degree (1971) in industrial engineering and operations research from the University of California, Berkeley.

Wing's primary research interest is in health workforce planning and policy-making. He has published numerous reports and articles on the supply and demand for health personnel, many in peer-reviewed journals.

Wing is also president of Planning and Research Services, Inc., a management consulting firm providing technical services to business and government.

Sabrina Wong completed her BSN at the University of British Columbia in 1992. In 1997 she completed a master's degree in community health nursing administration at the University of California, San Francisco, and entered UCSF's PhD nursing program.

Wong currently holds the position of Graduate Students Association president at UCSF. As head of student government, she is addressing interdisciplinary education, diversity, student participation in campus governance, and support services for students.

She has received the Outstanding Master of Science Student Award, as well as an award through the Williams and Wilkins Graduate Student Scholarship Competition.

Wong completed an internship at the UCSF Center for the Health Professions in 1996, where her responsibilities included assisting with the symposium at which initial drafts of the chapters of this book were presented.

To our colleagues at the
UCSF Center for the Health Professions

Strategies for the Future of Nursing

PART ONE

PAST, PRESENT, AND FUTURE

*Trends in Health Care and
the Nursing Workforce*

CHAPTER ONE

The Changing Health Care Environment

Edward O'Neil

In this first chapter, O'Neil argues that the challenges confronting nursing leaders in all quarters are a product of a fundamental realignment of the financial, organizational, and political structure of the United States's system of health care. He identifies six themes shaping the formation of this new system, and points to growing evidence that what will finally emerge is a system of care that is more managed, integrated, dependent upon evidence, and focused in the ambulatory or community-based setting than the current system. It will also make better use of information and communication technology and will place more emphasis on the psychosocial-behavioral dimensions of care and health. O'Neil believes that the emergent system will value those professions that understand these realities and incorporate them into patterns of practice. The nursing profession has a natural affinity in many of these domains and will find easy accommodation with others. The key to strategic success for the nursing profession is recognizing these strengths.

The 1990s have witnessed a dramatic transformation of the financing, organization, and delivery of health care in the United States. This transformation is, in turn, generating changes in the roles, responsibilities, and employment patterns of all health professionals. The effects of these changes are especially pronounced for registered nurses (RNs), who constitute the largest health care occupation in the country.

TRENDS IN HEALTH CARE DELIVERY IN THE UNITED STATES

The U.S. health care system is now undergoing the most significant transformation of this century. A familiar set of professional and institutional relationships among independent professional groups, independent nonprofit health care institutions, and public and private payers of heath care expenses is being rearranged rapidly. For most of this century these professional groups and institutions have dominated the structure of health care and have successfully kept it outside of both public-governmental and private-market mechanisms for governance. Though informed by both policy and the market, health care in America has been a fairly autonomous province for action by relatively independent professionals and institutions. This has fostered actions that seem counterintuitive to the workings of the market, such as increases in the price of services despite an oversupply of providers and the continued public subsidy of specialty training when signals indicate that an adequate number of these professionals have been trained.

Such arrangements for the organization, delivery, and financing of health care were appropriate as long as those who consumed its services—individuals and organizations—perceived it as in their interests to leave the system intact or were unwilling to pay the costs of realigning it to provide different outputs. Increasingly this does not seem to be the case. Purchasers, both public and private, continue to express their dissatisfaction with the cost of health care and its rate of growth. They also express concerns about standardization and quality measures used within the health care system. Public opinion polls suggest that the general public continues to be dissatisfied with the cost and value of the health care system. However, consumers retain high esteem for the individual health care providers with which they interact.

Added to these issues of cost and quality is the ongoing concern about access to care. National surveys estimate that forty-five million to sixty million individuals are without health insurance at some point each year and that the number is rising. Uninsured individuals are more likely to delay seeking care until their conditions become severe, which can increase the cost of treatment. Delays are especially problematic for uninsured individuals with communicable diseases. Gaps in health insurance coverage have contributed to increases in rates of tuberculosis and childhood diseases over the past fifteen years and have prevented some persons with HIV and AIDS from receiving the most effective, up-to-date treatment.

At many levels—individual and corporate, public and private—there are growing demands for change in health care. This dissatisfaction was the catalyst for the Clinton administration's Health Security Act of 1994 and other health care reform proposals. For a variety of reasons efforts to enact comprehensive legislative reforms failed, but the problems besetting the system of cost, quality, consumer satisfaction, and access remain. These forces are now coming together to move health care toward a more market-oriented system that responds to the needs of organized purchasers. This market movement is creating two additional market phenomena. The first is the wholesale transformation of health insurance companies into health plans or health companies providing products and services that meet the cost and quality standards of the organized purchasers. Second, and perhaps the more visible of the two, is the rapid consolidation of health care providers—hospitals, professional groups, other health care delivery assets, and others—into integrated systems of care. In many cases they also move from not-for-profit and public status into private, for-profit ownership. Some of these integrated systems incorporate the old health insurance entity along with the providers to create comprehensive systems of care.

These three markets—purchasers, plans, and providers—are working toward separate and often conflicting economic goals and are creating an enormous force for further consolidation and integration in health care. (See Chapter Four for a more detailed discussion of the evolution of health care markets.) The full meaning and implications of this transformation are unknown at this time, but certain trends are likely to characterize health care in the United States as we enter the twenty-first century. These trends, not just the linear extension of our current health care reality, offer the most important backdrop to any consideration of the future of nursing. A discussion of these trends follows.

More Integrated

One major cause of the excessive cost of care is the oversupply of both institutional providers and health professionals. Health care institutions and professionals have demonstrated little capacity to discipline themselves in terms of size or costs. In partial response to growing demands from purchasers for accountability for cost and quality, provider resources are increasingly linked through financial and other arrangements with the goal of streamlining services to reduce excess capacity. As these new systems struggle to perform they will also be forced to integrate their resources to organize and deliver care more effectively and efficiently. Because of the relatively high level of oversupply of providers, the incentive to integrate will be significant, with those providers who fail being increasingly marginal to the central action in health care.

More Intensively Managed

One is tempted to link integration and management; they certainly are products of the same forces in health care. But more intensive management will be a distinct product of the emerging integrated systems. Management will also be different. In the past, health care management existed to organize and deliver services around a logic and accountability that only made sense to the incumbents within the system. The few external standards were general and were not structured to provide detailed direction to the work of professionals and institutions. Much of the way the health care system was set up served the interests and needs of those incumbents—hospital administrators, physicians, nurses, and the like.

Certainly there was no external financial accountability and little consumer accountability. Quality was often defined and measured by those responsible for producing it, with little emphasis on patient outcomes or input from those outside the system. The emerging managerial structures will be focused on new system values of cost reduction, consumer satisfaction, and demonstrable quality. At least in the near term, management will place the highest priority on cost reduction. Consumer satisfaction and demonstrable quality will be important but will be addressed in a new framework in which cost considerations are paramount. An innovation will not only have to improve patient outcomes but do so cost-effectively. In other words, the emerging system will be more managed and focused on achieving different goals.

More Evidence Based

The current system of health care depends upon the unfettered and independent judgment of professionals, often working in isolation or without checks on their judgment. This is of course borne out of their capacity as specialists with expert knowledge and skills, but is also a by-product of the monopoly we give to health care providers to define and limit scope of practice. Recent research points to wide variation in the treatment of many diseases and conditions, even those for which studies have demonstrated that specific treatment regimens are the most cost-effective and efficacious. The new system will move some of that accountability from the individual professional to the system, and the system will increasingly demand evidence-based data about performance that can be weighed against objective standards of cost, quality, or satisfaction.

More Ambulatory or Community Based

The emerging system will place greater value on the delivery of individual services in physical locations where low cost and high quality and satisfaction can be achieved. Currently the system is moving as much care as possible out of high-cost hospital settings. It seems likely that this will continue, but that delivery of services in these settings will, out of necessity, have to meet the same evidence-based standards now being applied to hospitals.

More Emphasis on Information and Communications Technology

Information and communications technologies are revolutionizing most other service industries in the United States. The health care system has always made extensive use of information, but in a highly idiosyncratic manner with little effective management of emerging technology. However, this pattern appears to be changing as payers and providers seek to achieve new system goals. This technology is likely to be the single most important resource in the eventual reengineering of the core processes of health care, transforming both the clinical and nonclinical dimensions of care. It is also the mechanism by which more of the knowledge about the health care system will be made available to the patient and consumer in a more useful manner.

More Emphasis on the Psychosocial-Behavioral

The current health system remains focused on the biomedical dimensions of health care. This resulted from an orientation to disease and its relationship to health and a phenomenal array of technology invented in the twentieth century to treat these diseases or their implications. This orientation has led to many aspects of health care becoming radically reductionistic. Psychosocial-behavioral factors affecting health have often been dismissed or ignored. The emerging systems are more likely to ask questions about the efficacy and cost-effectiveness of an intervention, not whether it falls within the biomedical modality. This in turn will open new opportunities for those strategies to improve health or treat diseases that fall outside the traditional biomedical realm.

CONCLUSION

The ways we organize, deliver, and think about health care in the United States are rapidly changing. Integrated managed care–oriented systems have values different from those we associate with traditional fee-for-service health care. Our health care will become more managed, more technology based, more emphasizing of psychosocial behavioral dimensions, more evidence and outcome based, and more community oriented.

Each of the trends discussed in this chapter might rightly be the subject of an entire study, and many are featured in other chapters. Their identification here is intended to begin a discussion of the ongoing elements that will compose the future health care landscape which, in turn, will alter the roles, responsibilities, and employment patterns of registered nurses.

CHAPTER TWO

The Nursing Workforce and Nursing Education

An Overview of Trends

Janet Coffman
Noelle Blick
Sabrina Wong

Projecting nursing's future requires understanding both the health care environment and the current state of the nursing profession. The authors provide a broad overview of trends in registered nurses' (RNs') demographic characteristics, employment patterns, and educational attainment. As the health care system has expanded over the past five decades, so has the size of the RN workforce, but it remains a workforce in which racial minorities and males are underrepresented, and appears to be aging faster than the rest of the professional workforce. Although the nursing profession has moved somewhat out of the hospital setting, nearly two out of three nurses remain in that setting, and their future employment patterns depend on what strategies hospitals pursue and how successful they are in that pursuit. Hospital-based diploma programs once dominated the educational scene but have now all but disappeared. The past twenty years have seen phenomenal growth in the associate-level training that now is the predominant pathway to entry-level practice in nursing. These same two decades have witnessed significant growth in advanced-level training for nursing professionals. The information presented in this chapter grounds the discussion of nursing's future in subsequent chapters.

The implications of the transformation of health care in the United States described in Chapter One are increasingly evident in trends in registered nurse employment. This chapter provides an overview of recent trends in RN employment and education. Although the majority of RNs continue to be employed in hospitals, jobs are shifting to other settings. Analysis of trends in RN education suggest too few RNs have bachelor's or advanced degrees to meet projected future requirements. Assessment of demographic trends reveals significant changes in the age distribution of RNs and a large gap between the percentage of racial and ethnic minorities among RNs and those in the population as a whole. This chapter addresses current characteristics of the RN workforce, providing a foundation for the discussion of future trends in supply and demand for RNs in Chapter Three.

SUPPLY AND CHARACTERISTICS OF REGISTERED NURSES

Nursing is the largest of the health professions, and RNs far outnumber the other two categories of nursing personnel (licensed practical and vocational nurses and unlicensed nursing aides and assistants). According to the National Sample Survey of Registered Nurses, the most detailed and systematic source of data about RNs in the United States, an estimated 2.6 million RNs were licensed to practice in the United States in 1996 (Moses, 1997). The number of RNs has risen steadily over the past thirty years, and the rate of growth has outstripped that of the U.S. population as a whole. Between 1980 and 1994 the number of RNs per 100,000 population in the U.S. increased by 40 percent. (See Figure 3.1 in Chapter Three for a graphical display of trends in RN employment.)

Analysis of RNs' demographic characteristics reveal other important trends in the RN workforce. The gender, racial-ethnic, and age distributions of RNs differ significantly from those of the U.S. adult population as a whole. The most dramatic disparity concerns gender. Nursing has always been a predominantly female occupation. Although the number of male RNs has grown significantly in recent years, men still account for a very small percentage of RNs. Estimates derived from the 1996 National Sample Survey indicate that 94.6 percent of RNs are women and 5.4 percent are men (Moses, 1997).

Also, all racial and ethnic minorities except Asian and Pacific Islanders remain underrepresented among RNs. According to preliminary data from the 1996 survey, only 9.7 percent of RNs in the United States are racial or ethnic minorities (Moses, 1997). In contrast, estimates by the U.S. Bureau of Census (1995) indicate that in 1992 nonwhites accounted for 24 percent of all U.S. residents. African Americans comprise 11 percent of U.S. residents but only 4.2 percent of registered nurses. Similarly, 9 percent of U.S. residents are Hispanic but only 1.6 percent of RNs are Hispanic.

The percentage of racial and ethnic minorities in the U.S. population is increasing and is expected to rise to 38 percent by 2025 (U.S. Bureau of the Census, 1995). The RN population will remain less diverse than the population as a whole for the foreseeable future unless the number of racial and ethnic minorities completing RN education programs increases dramatically.

A third difference between the RN workforce and the population as a whole concerns age distribution. The average age of RNs has increased steadily over the past twenty years. Figure 2.1 shows the trend in the age distribution of RNs from 1980 to 1996. The rise in the average age of RNs cannot be explained solely by changes in the age distribution of the professionals in the U.S. labor force as a whole. In fact, the age distribution of RNs differs markedly from that of all professional workers. The number of employed RNs under age thirty decreased 20 percent between 1988 and 1992, whereas the percentage of all

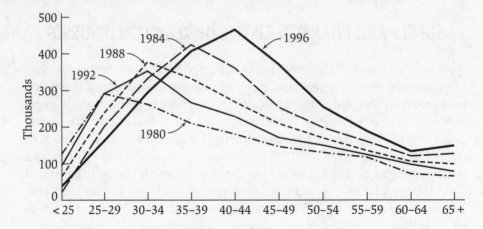

Figure 2.1. Age Distribution of the Registered Nurse Population, 1980–1992.
Source: Moses, 1997

workers under age thirty decreased only 8 percent (National Advisory Council on Nursing Education and Practice, 1996). The average age at which RNs enter practice has increased, suggesting that this difference in age distribution will continue for the foreseeable future.

CURRENT RN EMPLOYMENT PATTERNS

How many RNs are actually working as RNs? How are they dispersed across health care settings? Are RNs who have certain levels of education more likely to be employed in nursing or in particular settings? This section seeks to answer these and other questions regarding current RN employment patterns. Projections of supply and demand for RNs in the twenty-first century are discussed in detail in Chapter Three.

Employment in Nursing

Over the past decade, the rate of growth in RN employment has been much greater than those of all other occupations. Data from the Census Bureau's current population survey indicate that between 1983 and 1994 RN employment grew by 30 percent whereas employment in all other occupations grew only by an average of 16 percent (Buerhaus and Staiger, 1996). This aggregate growth in RN employment was accompanied by a large increase in the percentage of RNs working in their profession. According to the National Sample Survey of Registered Nurses, only 77 percent of RNs were employed in nursing in 1980 (Moses, 1994). By 1996, that had risen to 83 percent (Moses, 1997).

Among RNs working in nursing, the percentages employed on a full- and part-time basis remained relatively stable from 1980 to 1984. Roughly two-thirds worked full-time and one-third worked part-time (Moses, 1994). However, during the period from 1984 to 1996 the percentage of all RNs who were employed full-time increased sharply from 52 to 59 percent (Moses, 1997). Buerhaus's (1993, 1995) research suggests that the initial increase may have been a short-term result of the recession, perhaps having led some RNs to temporarily switch from part- to full-time employment to compensate for loss of income from unemployed partners. However, this trend continues today despite robust economic growth.

Employment by Major Setting

Hospitals remain the largest employer of RNs in the United States, but employment opportunities are gradually shifting to other sectors. As Figure 2.2 shows, the National Sample Survey data indicate that hospitals employed 60 percent of RNs employed in nursing in 1996 (Moses, 1997). This percentage represented a significant decrease from the 1992 National Sample Survey, which estimated that 67 percent of RNs employed in nursing were employed in the hospital setting (Moses, 1994).

Among nonhospital settings, community-public health nursing was the only arena to experience a large increase in RN employment during this period. The percentage of RNs employed in community–public health settings rose from 10 to 13 percent, paralleling the rapid expansion of home care during this five-year period (Moses, 1997). Despite the dramatic shift in the delivery of many health care services from inpatient to ambulatory settings, employment of RNs in

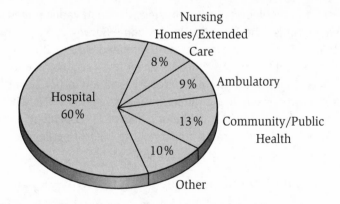

Figure 2.2. Registered Nurses by Employment Setting, 1996.
Source: Moses, 1997

ambulatory settings (excluding hospital outpatient departments) grew only slightly, rising from 7 to 8.1 percent of employed RNs.

The large growth of enrollment in managed care plans is affecting demand for RNs. Buerhaus and Staiger found that since 1992 there has been a small but steady increase in the percentage of RNs employed in home care and other non-hospital settings (Buerhaus and Staiger, 1996). This shift has been most evident in states with high rates of enrollment in HMOs. In addition, employment of RNs increased at a slower rate in states with high HMO enrollment. These findings suggest that sectoral shifts in the RN labor market will become more pronounced at the national level as HMO enrollment increases in states where current enrollment rates are low.

However, over the past decade, changes in hospital staffing patterns have mitigated the shift of RN employment to nonhospital settings. Aiken, Sochalski, and Anderson (1996) found that employment of RN personnel in hospitals increased between 1982 and 1993 despite a significant drop in hospital utilization. In contrast, employment of LPNs and LVNs and unlicensed nursing personnel declined, suggesting that hospitals substituted RNs for other nursing personnel as changes in reimbursement and technology precipitated an increase in patient acuity. Whether this trend will continue into the twenty-first century remains unclear, though some experts believe it will reverse as hospitals face increasing pressure to control costs.

In addition, the rapid expansion of hospital outpatient services resulted in many RNs merely shifting from inpatient to outpatient departments within hospitals (Wunderlich, Sloan, and Davis, 1996). The number of RNs working in hospital outpatient departments rose by over 100 percent between 1988 and 1996 (Moses, 1994, 1997). Many of these RNs work in outpatient units that perform surgical procedures and other services that previously were available only on an inpatient basis.

The mix of RNs by highest level of nursing education varies somewhat across employment settings. The 1996 National Sample Survey of Registered Nurses indicates that in 1996 nursing homes and extended care facilities employed a much higher percentage of RNs whose highest level of nursing education was a diploma or associate degree (74.1 percent) than any other setting. Student health services settings employed the largest percentages of RNs whose highest level of nursing education was a bachelor's degree (39.5 percent). Not surprisingly, nursing education programs employed the highest percentage (75.1 percent) of RNs with graduate degrees in nursing (Moses, 1997).

The Role of Advanced Practice Nurses

In recent years, policymakers and health care delivery systems have focused increased attention on the role of advanced practice nurses (APNs). Although APNs accounted for only 6.3 percent of all RNs in the United States in 1996

(Moses, 1997), their numbers are increasing rapidly. The number of RNs interested in pursuing training in advanced practice has increased significantly and APN education programs have expanded to meet this demand. Some experts have speculated that the growth of enrollment in managed care plans will lead to increased utilization of APNs, as they can provide many of the same services as physicians at lower cost, at least in terms of salary and benefits, often achieving better patient compliance and satisfaction.

The National Sample Survey of Registered Nurses indicates that in 1996 an estimated 161,712 nurses had formal preparation for practice as APNs, of whom 74,882 (46 percent) work in positions with APN job titles. Most APNs are educated as either clinical nurse specialists (53,799) or nurse practitioners (63,191). There are considerably fewer nurse anesthetists (30,386) and nurse midwives (6,534) (Moses, 1997). Most nurse practitioners are prepared as primary care providers, whereas clinical nurse specialists generally focus on a specific specialty. Approximately 65 percent of nurse practitioners graduating in 1995 were prepared as family, adult, or pediatric nurse practitioners (National League for Nursing, 1997).

RN EDUCATION

The other chapters in this anthology raise many questions regarding future demand for RNs. Fralic, Bellack, and Bauman project growing demand for RNs prepared at the baccalaureate and graduate levels and declining demand for associate degree- and diploma-prepared RNs in their respective chapters on demand for RNs in hospital, ambulatory, and home care settings. Authors repeatedly cite market pressures likely to increase demand for APNs. Yet Gilliss and Mundinger conclude in Chapter Nine that competition from specialist physicians may constrain demand for APNs. Harrington's assessment of the long-term care industry in Chapter Six suggests that low reimbursement rates and pressure to maximize profits will constrain employment of APNs in long-term care settings despite their documented ability to improve the quality of care residents receive. In addition, a number of authors, most notably Fralic, question the appropriateness of current patterns of age distribution among RN students.

Whatever the future holds for RNs, nursing's ability to meet future demand will hinge in large part on the adequacy of the current infrastructure for nursing education and the characteristics of the students educated. This section describes current trends in nursing education and the characteristics of nursing students.

Distribution of RNs by Educational Level

RNs may be classified into roughly five groups with respect to the highest level of education they have completed.

- Associate degree (two-year program based at a community college)
- Diploma (three-year program based at a hospital)
- Baccalaureate degree (four-year program based at a four-year college)
- Master's degree (one- to two-year graduate program)
- Doctoral degree

RNs can enter nursing education at any of these levels and subsequently return to school to pursue further education in nursing. Many nursing schools educating RNs at the bachelor's level have developed "RN to BSN" programs that are tailored to the educational needs of RNs who already have a diploma or associate degree. A small number of master's entry programs target persons with bachelor's degrees in nonnursing fields. Most APN education programs are master's programs that require a bachelor's degree in nursing or another field as a prerequisite for admission, although some APNs continue to be educated in certificate programs that admit RNs who have only a diploma or associate degree. A growing number of nursing schools offer post-master's certificate programs in ARN specialties for RNs who already have master's degrees. In addition, some nursing schools have developed "RN to MSN" programs that enable associate degree nurses to complete a master's degree without first obtaining a bachelor's degreee.

Trends in nursing education are displayed graphically in Figure 3.2 in Chapter Three. Data compiled by the National League for Nursing (1996) reveal that the number of RNs graduating from basic nursing education programs each year increased by 41 percent from the 1973–74 to the 1994–95 academic year, rising from 67,061 to 97,052 graduates per year. Graduations will fall off slightly over the next several years, due to a slight (2 percent) decrease in the number of new students admitted, from 129,897 in 1993–94 to 127,184 in 1994–95.

Since the 1940s, many nursing leaders have recommended that a baccalaureate degree be the minimum level of education required for practice as an RN (Friss, 1994). Progress toward this goal has been quite slow, due to the absence of state laws mandating the bachelor's degree for entry to practice and the lack of significant differentials in salaries and employment opportunities. Three-quarters of RNs continue to receive their basic nursing education through diploma or associate degree programs. The 1997 National Sample Survey of RNs revealed that 36 percent of RNs in the United States in 1997 had received their basic nursing education from diploma programs, 38 percent from associate degree programs, and 26 percent from bachelor's degree programs (Moses, 1997).

This finding reflects two factors. First, many RNs in practice today completed their basic nursing education prior to the decline in enrollment in diploma programs that began in the 1970s. Although diploma programs accounted for only 7 percent of basic nursing graduates in 1995 (National League for Nursing,

1996), approximately 32 percent of all RNs who completed their basic RN education prior to 1977 graduated from diploma programs (Moses, 1994).

Second, associate degree programs graduate more RNs per year than bachelor's degree programs, and the number of graduations from associate degree programs has risen faster than the number from baccalaureate degree programs. The latter increased 84 percent between the 1973–74 and 1994–95 academic years (from 16,957 to 31,254), but that increase was not sufficient to keep pace with the 103 percent increase in the number of graduates from associate degree programs during that period (28,919 to 58,749) (National League for Nursing, 1995, 1996). Thus, the last twenty-five years have witnessed primarily a shift from diploma to associate degree programs as the main source of new RNs with only a relatively modest increase in the percentage of new RNs educated at the baccalaureate level.

The percentage of RNs educated at baccalaureate and master's levels has increased over the years, but a large gap remains between the ideal and the actual distribution of RNs by educational attainment (see Figure 2.3). According to the 1996 National Sample Survey of RNs, the highest level of education attained by 58.4 percent of registered nurses was either a diploma (23.8 percent) or an associate degree (34.6 percent) in nursing. An estimated 31.8 percent had received bachelor's degrees in nursing or a related field. RNs holding master's degrees accounted for 9.1 percent and doctoral degree holders for 0.6 percent of RNs (Moses, 1997).

RNs who complete their basic nursing education in diploma or associate degree programs can obtain bachelor's degrees in nursing through programs sponsored by four-year colleges that are commonly referred to as "RN to BSN" programs. Approximately 14 percent of graduates of associate degree programs and 21 percent of graduates of diploma programs later obtain at least a baccalaureate degree

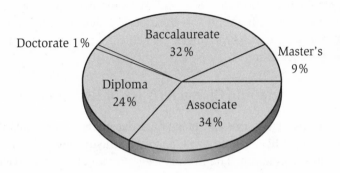

Figure 2.3. Registered Nurses by Highest Level of Nursing Education, 1996.
Source: Moses, 1997.

in nursing (National Advisory Council on Nursing Education and Practice, 1996). According to the National League for Nursing (1996), 11,995 RNs graduated from RN to BSN programs during the 1994–95 academic year. Graduations from these programs have increased significantly in recent years, with a 19 percent increase between the 1992–93 and 1994–95 academic years. However, graduations have yet to reach a level at which they will significantly increase the percentage of RNs with bachelor's degrees.

Enrollment in and graduations from master's degree programs in nursing— the most common pathway to advanced practice—has soared over the past twenty years. According to the National League for Nursing (1997), the number of graduations from master's degree programs of all types rose by 246 percent from 1974–75 to 1994–95, rising from 2,678 to 9,261 per year. Such graduations will continue to rise for the next several years, due in large part to the large increase in the number of students enrolled in nurse practitioner programs between 1993 and 1995. According to surveys conducted by the National Organization of Nurse Practitioner Faculties (Harper and Johnson, 1996), the number of students enrolled in nurse practitioner programs has more than doubled, rising from 2,812 in 1993 to 7,926 in 1995.

The historical enrollment patterns of students in RN to BSN and graduate programs suggest that nursing educators may have difficulty rapidly expanding the numbers of RNs educated at baccalaureate and master's levels. Most students enroll in these programs on a part-time basis. Data published by the American Association of Colleges of Nursing (Berlin, Bednash, and Scott, 1997) indicate that during the 1996–97 academic year, 86 percent of students in RN to BSN programs were enrolled on a part-time basis. In 1995 part-time students accounted for roughly 64 percent of nurse practitioner students and 74 percent of clinical nurse specialist students (National League for Nursing, 1997). The number of master's degree students enrolled each year on a part-time basis has risen dramatically since 1980, whereas the number enrolled full-time has been relatively stable. If demand for BSNs and APNs increases as some experts predict, nursing schools will not be able to respond quickly to projected increases in demand for BSNs and APNs unless the percentage of students enrolled full-time increases significantly.

Demographic Characteristics of RN Students

Several of the chapters in this anthology raise questions about the consequences of current trends in RN age and racial and ethnic distribution on nursing's ability to meet future demand. The average age at graduation from basic nursing education has increased dramatically since the mid-1970s. According to the National Sample Survey, the average age at graduation for RNs graduating prior to 1976 was 22.7. In contrast, for RNs graduating between 1991 and 1996 the average had risen to 31.7 (Moses, 1997). The rise in the average age of RN students reflects broader trends in enrollment in higher education as well as the infusion of individuals seeking second careers as RNs. Among recent graduates of basic RN programs, 32 percent were originally educated as licensed practical or vocational nurses (LPNs or LVNs) or attained academic degrees in nonnursing fields (National Advisory Council on Nursing Education and Practice, 1996).

Associate degree students graduating between 1991 and 1996 were considerably older at graduation than their peers in diploma and baccalaureate programs. Associate degree graduates were an average of 33.5 years of age at graduation versus 31.1 years for diploma graduates and 28.0 years for baccalaureate graduates (Figure 2.4) (Moses, 1997). The high average age of graduates of associate degree programs is of particular interest given that 61 percent of all RNs graduating from basic nursing programs between the 1990–91 and 1994–95 academic years graduated from associate degree programs (National League for Nursing, 1996).

Similarly, current trends in the number of racial and ethnic minority students enrolled in basic nursing education programs are not likely to alter significantly the racial and ethnic composition of the RN workforce. As with practicing RNs the percentage of whites among graduates of basic RN programs is considerably higher than the 76 percent of whites in the U.S. population as a whole in 1992 (U.S. Bureau of the Census, 1995). Among students graduating from basic RN programs between the 1989–90 and 1993–94 academic years, whites accounted for at least 86 percent of students in basic nursing programs at each level. Baccalaureate programs enrolled a slightly higher percentage of racial and ethnic minority students (14 percent) than diploma (11.2 percent) and associate degree programs (13.3 percent). Racial and ethnic minorities are even less well repre-

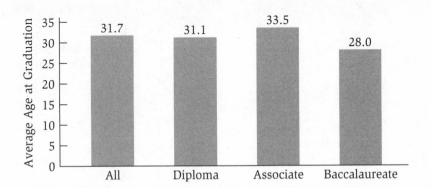

Figure 2.4. Average Age at Graduation from Basic Nursing Education Programs, Average for Graduations Between 1991 and 1996.

Source: Moses, 1997

sented among nursing students at the graduate level. According to the National League for Nursing (1997), during the 1994–95 academic year 88 percent of recipients of master's degrees in nursing were white.

The racial and ethnic composition of recent graduates of basic RN programs stands in marked contrast to that of recent graduates of LPN and LVN programs. As Figure 2.5 illustrates, during the period from the 1990–91 to the 1994–95 academic year, blacks accounted for much larger shares of LPN and LVN graduates than of basic RN graduates. Blacks accounted for over twice as high a percentage of LPN and LVN graduates (15 percent) than of basic RN graduates (7 percent). Indeed, blacks are a larger percentage of LPN and LVN graduates than of the U.S. population in 1992 as a whole.

CONCLUSION

Although the rapid pace of change in the health care industry renders precise projections impossible, this chapter suggests several likely developments in RN education and employment. First, although hospitals may continue to employ more RNs than any other setting, jobs will increasingly shift to other sectors. Future levels of RN employment in hospitals will depend in large part on prevailing hospital staffing patterns. If hospitals reduce excess capacity and sub-

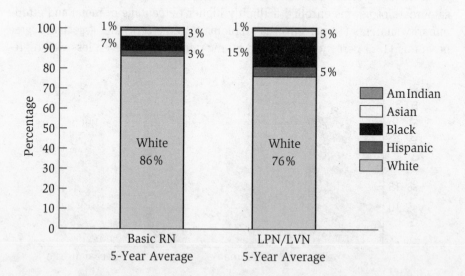

Figure 2.5. Basic RN and LPN/LVN Graduates by Race/Ethnicity, Average from 1990–91 to 1994–95.

Source: National League for Nursing, 1997.

stitute non-RNs for RNs wherever possible, aggregate employment of RNs in hospitals may well decline unless demand for RNs in other sectors increases enough to absorb those displaced.

However, the biggest challenge facing nursing is educating RNs for their emerging roles. As Bellack and Bauman discuss in detail in Chapters Seven and Eight, respectively, practice in nonhospital settings requires more autonomy and greater emphasis on health promotion. RNs in supervisory roles will need both managerial and teaching skills. Yet over 50 percent of all RNs have been educated solely in diploma and associate degree programs that historically have not emphasized competencies in these areas. Strong partnerships among educators, employers, and communities will be needed to develop effective approaches to bridge the apparent gap between RNs' competencies and employers' expectations.

References

Aiken, L. H., Sochalski, J., and Anderson, G. F. "Downsizing the Hospital Nursing Workforce." *Health Affairs*, 1996, *15*(4), 88–92.

American Hospital Association. *National Hospital Survey: Special Supplemental Survey.* Chicago: American Hospital Association, 1995.

Berlin, L. E., Bednash, G. D., and Scott, D. L. *1996–97 Enrollments and Graduations in Baccalaureate and Graduate Programs in Nursing.* Washington, D.C.: American Association of Colleges of Nursing, 1997.

Buerhaus, P. I. "Effects of RN Wages and Non-Wage Income on the Performance of the Hospital RN Labor Market." *Nursing Economics,* 1993, *11*(3), 129–135.

Buerhaus, P. I. "Economic Pressure Building in the Employed RN Labor Market." *Nursing Economics,* 1995, *13*(3), 137–141.

Buerhaus, P. I., and Staiger, D. O. "Managed Care and the Nurse Labor Market." *Journal of the American Medical Association,* 1996, *276*(18), 1487–1493.

Friss, L. "Nursing Studies Laid End to End Form a Circle." *Journal of Health Politics, Policy, and Law,* 1994, *19*(3), 597–631.

Harper, J., and Johnson, J. *NONPF Workforce Policy Project Technical Report: Nurse Practitioner Education Programs 1988–1995.* Washington D.C.: National Organization of Nurse Practitioner Faculties, 1996.

Moses, E. B. *The Registered Nurse Population: Findings from the National Sample Survey of Registered Nurses, March 1992.* Rockville, Md.: Division of Nursing, U.S. Bureau of Health Professions, Health Resources and Services Administration, Public Health Service, U.S. Department of Health and Human Services, 1994.

Moses, E. B. *The Registered Nurse Population: Findings from the National Sample Survey of Registered Nurses, March 1996.* Rockville, Md.: Division of Nursing, U.S. Bureau of Health Professions, Health Resources and Services Administration, Public Health Service, U.S. Department of Health and Human Services, 1997.

National Advisory Council on Nursing Education and Practice. *Report to the Secretary of Health and Human Services on the Basic Registered Nurse Workforce.* Washington, D.C.: U.S. Department of Health and Human Services, 1996.

National League for Nursing. *Nursing Datasource 1995.* New York: National League for Nursing Press, 1995.

National League for Nursing. *Nursing Datasource 1996.* New York: National League for Nursing Press, 1996.

National League for Nursing. *Nursing Data Review 1997.* New York: National League for Nursing Press, 1997.

U.S. Bureau of the Census. *Statistical Abstract of the United States 1995.* Washington, D.C.: U.S. Bureau of the Census, 1995.

Wunderlich, G. S., Sloan, F. A., and Davis, C. K. (eds.). *Nursing Staff in Hospitals and Nursing Homes: Is It Adequate?* Washington, D.C.: National Academy Press, 1996.

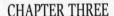

CHAPTER THREE

Projecting the Future Supply and Demand for Registered Nurses

Edward Salsberg
Paul Wing
Carol S. Brewer

As the changes in the health care system outlined in Chapter One progress, they will alter the pattern of demand for nursing professionals. Nursing is the largest single profession in health care, and, as discussed in Chapter Two, the number of nurses has grown consistently with the overall expansion of health care over the past five decades. However, health care is now undergoing fundamental structural changes that will likely alter the cyclical pattern of nursing oversupply and shortage that has characterized nursing in the past. The more significant elements of this transformation are decreased use of hospitals, fewer but higher-acuity admissions, shorter lengths of stay, consolidation and downsizing of hospitals, movement of care to ambulatory settings, competition with other providers, new technologies, and alteration of the processes for the delivery of care in the inpatient settings. Increased competition among health care providers will serve to drive the transition along at a much faster pace than would typically be expected in health care. This complex mix of factors combines to produce the following projections: a significant growth in demand in the immediate future for advanced practice nurses; a reduction in demand for RNs over the next ten to fifteen years; and a growth in demand for unlicensed assistive personnel, who are supervised by RNs. Whether this situation will produce an oversupply of RNs is heavily dependent upon how well leaders in nursing education understand and respond to these trends. In particular, nursing educators must closely monitor class size in the associate and diploma levels and not overreact to the current growth in demand for advance practice nurses.

Predicting the future demand for nurses in the United States during this time of rapid evolution in health care financing and delivery is particularly important but very difficult. Producing too few nurses or the wrong skill mix can diminish quality of care, create gaps in service, and result in inefficiencies. Producing too many nurses wastes society's educational investment and is unfair to individual graduates who cannot find employment commensurate with their education.

Although it is difficult to predict the exact changes in supply and demand (particularly their magnitude and timing), general directions for the nursing workforce are discernible. The trends in health care outlined in Chapter One are expected to increase the demand for advance practice nurses, limit the growth in demand for registered nurses, and increase job opportunities for unlicensed assistive personnel. Whether there will be surpluses or shortages of nurses depends in part on how the supply side (nursing schools and prospective students) responds to changes in demand. This chapter reviews the following:

- Current trends in the supply and demand for nurses
- Recent changes in health care and other factors that are likely to influence the supply and demand for nurses
- Recent studies and predictions
- The authors' predictions and observations on future supply and demand
- The implications of these predictions for nursing education

The chapter focuses on "demand" rather than "need" for nurses. Demand is an economic concept that assumes that the health care system responds to a variety of factors to determine how many of what types of nurses to use in providing services. Although patients have needs, these can often be met in a number of ways by a number of different types of workers. Demand for a specific profession or occupation reflects how the health care system has chosen to meet those needs in light of a variety of factors, including supply, salary level, licensing and other regulatory requirements, availability of alternatives, and other factors.

The focus of this chapter is registered nurses, who compose the single largest component of the nursing profession. However, because other nurses also play an important role in determining the demand and roles of RNs, the chapter briefly discusses other nursing personnel as well.

THE CURRENT NURSING WORKFORCE

There are several important sources of data about the nursing workforce and nursing education in the United States:

- The Division of Nursing (DN) of the U.S. Department of Health and Human Services. DN collects extensive information about the demographic and practice characteristics of registered nurses every four years. DN tabulations are generally based on headcounts, one per nurse.

- The Bureau of Labor Statistics (BLS). BLS collects information on all kinds of employees, including several types of nurses, in all kinds of employment settings every three years. BLS data are generally counts of paychecks, which means that people holding down two jobs are counted twice.

- The American Hospital Association (AHA). AHA annually collects data on the numbers of full-time equivalent (FTE) RNs, as well as LPNs and LVNs, employed in several types of hospitals across the country. The FTE counts are generally lower than the headcount numbers in the DN reports and the paycheck numbers in the BLS reports.

- Information about nursing education programs (including admissions, enrollments, and graduates) is compiled annually by the National League for Nursing (NLN) and the American Association of Colleges of Nursing (AACN).

Unfortunately, lack of common time frames, standard definitions, and categories make comparisons, aggregations, and analysis of these data sets difficult. It is often impossible to link details from one of the sources with those of another. Nevertheless, some general patterns are evident.

As noted in Chapter Two, the overall supply of nurses has grown substantially over the past decade. Figure 3.1 shows that the number of RNs grew by

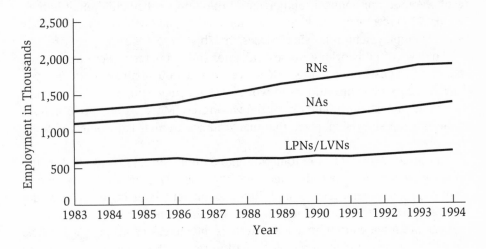

Figure 3.1. Nursing Employment in the United States (in Thousands) 1983 to 1994.

Source: U.S. Bureau of Labor Statistics, 1995

more than 46 percent between 1983 and 1994. The numbers of licensed practical and vocational nurses and nurse aides also grew over this period, but at a lesser rate—18 and 19 percent, respectively (Wunderlich, Sloan, and Davis, 1996). In 1994 there were a total of 1.9 million RNs, 702,000 LPNs and LVNs, and 1.4 million nurse and psychiatric aides.

A few caveats should be kept in mind when interpreting these data. The total reported for LPNs and LVNs may overstate their actual supply, because many RNs obtain certification or licensure as LPNs or LVNs to secure employment while they are in school. In addition, data on nurse aides do not encompass all unlicensed nursing personnel. Missing are a new category of multiskilled workers who perform a limited number of specific patient care tasks along with a variety of ancillary tasks. Anecdotal reports suggest employment of these workers is expanding rapidly.

LABOR FORCE PARTICIPATION RATES

The total "active nursing workforce" reflects the number of nurses that are licensed and employed in nursing. An understanding of current RN labor force participation trends is essential to projecting future supply. The labor force participation rate of RNs (that is, the percentage of nurses actively working as nurses) reached a plateau in 1996 at 82.7 percent after increasing an average of 0.5 percent each year since 1980 (Moses, 1997b). Of those RNs not working in nursing in 1996 who were neither seeking a nursing position nor working in a nonnursing occupation, over half were more than sixty years old; only 15 percent were forty or younger (86 percent of these nurses had children at home); almost 27 percent were working in nonnursing jobs, and 8 percent were actively seeking employment in nursing (Moses, 1997b).

Analysis of nonworking nurses indicates that 70 percent were working in nursing five years prior to the 1996 survey year. Of those nurses not employed in 1995, 22.1 percent returned to work in 1996, suggesting that there is considerable movement in and out of the workforce (Moses, 1997b, p. 68). This pattern is not surprising, given that many nurses are married women of childbearing age.

Our analysis of data from four National Sample Surveys conducted by the Division of Nursing shows that between 1980 and 1992, approximately 16 percent of RNs between ages fifty and fifty-nine left active nursing practice, as did 8 percent of forty- to forty-nine-year-olds. If these patterns persist, the increasing age of RNs at entry to practice as well as the increasing average age of RNs suggest the overall labor force participation rate of RNs may decrease in the coming years.

FACTORS INFLUENCING THE DEMAND FOR NURSES

Many factors influence the demand for nurses. Three are especially important in this era: changing health care organization and financing, changing population demographics, and new technologies in health care delivery.

Changes in the Organization of Health Care Services

The changes in the health care system described subsequently will have a major impact on the demand for nurses in the future. All of these changes are rooted in the broad trends in the U.S. health care system outlined in Chapter One and the evolution of health care markets described in Chapter Four. Chief among these changes will be decreased use of hospitals. There are strong pressures from all payers to reduce the use of hospitals, one of the most expensive sources of care and the setting with the largest number of nurses. Following are descriptions of the specific drivers of the decrease in hospital use.

Fewer Admissions. More and more services are being shifted to ambulatory settings. Primary care gatekeepers and more aggressive utilization review are also decreasing hospital use. However, patients who are admitted may be sicker and require more intensive care.

Shorter Lengths of Stay. Most hospitals across the nation are implementing strategies to move patients through the hospital more expeditiously. The strategies include preadmission testing, clinical pathways, case managers, and early discharge planning.

Hospital Consolidation and Downsizing. As hospital admissions and length of stay decline, the net number of patient days is likely to drop sharply. As hospitals merge and networks develop, some older hospitals will probably close altogether or be used for other purposes, such as ambulatory care or long-term care, which require less intensive RN staffing.

Reengineering and Substitution of Lower-Cost Personnel. Pressures to contain costs have created incentives for all types of health care facilities to find ways to use workers more efficiently. Substitution of lower-cost workers for higher-cost workers is a strategy used by many health care organizations across the country.

This strategy constitutes a major departure from past RN staffing patterns. Evidence prior to 1993 suggests that RNs were substituted for other kinds of nursing personnel (Aiken, Sochalski, and Anderson, 1996, p. 89). Since 1993, however, the pattern has changed, with lower-cost personnel being substituted for RNs. Data from the AHA National Hospital Panel Survey from 1993 to 1996 showed annual percentage changes in RN FTEs of –0.8 percent, –1.4 percent, and –0.2 percent, reversing years of positive growth (Ferguson, 1997). The slower growth of RN positions in hospitals, combined with decreasing patient length of stay and a likely continuation of increasing intensity of care, contributes to RNs' continuing concern over declining RN employment (Spetz, 1996, p. 18).

Competition in All Settings. Regardless of the setting, competition is likely to exert pressure to minimize costs. As hospitals, HMOs, health centers, and physician practices streamline operations to reduce costs and maintain market share, they typically reduce staff, including nurses. These practices are now being implemented in nursing homes and home care, as well.

The Aging of the Population

One of the major forces likely to increase future demand for all types of health care personnel is the aging of the population of the United States. There is little doubt that over the next three to five decades services to the elderly, including long-term care, will become a much larger component of the entire health care spectrum. The aging of the population and the increased rate of survival and longevity of individuals with chronic illnesses could add significantly to the responsibilities of the health care system. However, a major increase in the demand for health care and nursing personnel due to the aging of the population is not expected to lead to a large increase in demand for health care services and nursing personnel for the next ten or fifteen years.

In fact, the rate of increase in the numbers of people sixty-five and older will be at the lowest rate in U.S. history in the coming decade, reflecting the very low birth rates during the Depression and World War II. Although persons over sixty-five use more services than younger adults, the sharp rise in health care use rates and costs occur later, particularly for those over seventy-five. Thus, though the "baby boom" generation will begin to reach age sixty-five in 2010, its impact on the health care system will not be felt until 2020 when large numbers of people begin to reach seventy-five.

New Technologies

Tremendous investments are being made to identify, create, and design new technologies and medical advances to improve health and increase life expectancy. Genetic engineering companies are now joining pharmaceutical companies in an aggressive search for profitable new products to help treat and prevent diseases. It is likely that some (perhaps even many) of these efforts will ultimately result in successful new products and services. Over the next ten to twenty years, these advances are likely to reduce use of health facilities. In the past, most of the new technological developments were designed to improve the outcomes and effectiveness of care. However, with expanded competition in health care there is a growing investment in technologies designed specifically to reduce costs and increase efficiency.

Assessing the impact of any such innovations on nursing personnel is very difficult. Presumably, a new treatment or technology that reduces the incidence of disease or condition is likely to reduce the demand for health care in the short run. However, health care needs in later years resulting from increases in longevity may eventually offset some of the initial reductions. For example, a successful treatment for heart disease may ultimately result in a longer life expectancy but with significant increases in other chronic illnesses. However, new technologies and interventions that permit care on an ambulatory rather than inpatient basis could permanently reduce demand for nurses. Policymakers and health profession educators must be prepared for significant changes and must regularly reassess projections of demand and need for nursing services.

Other Factors That May Influence the Demand for RNs

A number of trends in other segments of the health care system could significantly affect these patterns and trends. Although changes like those described hereafter are expected to begin to take shape over the next decade, the recommendations presented assume that none will progress far enough to upset the basic equilibria that now exist in the health care system and health workforce.

Rationing of Health Care. Rationing could reduce the volume of services provided by the health care system. Our recommendations assume some reduction in service levels, especially in hospitals, but not drastic reductions.

Increased Use of Preventive Health Care and Self-Care. The greater emphasis on prevention and self-care could result in significant reduction in overall demand for institutional health care services of certain types, while increasing the demand for assistance with preventive care and self-care. Such trends could increase demand for RNs dramatically, if RNs are involved in coordinating, supervising, or teaching these care modalities.

Projecting Future Demand for Nurses

Four recent studies and reports forecast the future demand for RNs in the United States. The studies of the Bureau of Labor Statistics and the Division of Nursing are based on historical, quantitative data about the RN workforce.

Bureau of Labor Statistics (BLS) Labor Force Projections. The BLS is the leading source of official government projections of employment, wages, and other labor force statistics. The agency generates forecasts of future employment using a model that incorporates national demographic and economic trends, particularly industrial output. In November 1995, under its "moderate" assumptions, BLS projected an increase of 25 percent between 1994 and 2005, with a total of 2.4 million RNs employed in 2005, an increase of 473,000 over 1994 (U.S. Bureau of Labor Statistics, 1995, p. 66).

Bureau of Health Professions, Division of Nursing: General Services Demand Model. The General Services Demand Model (GSDM), developed by Vector Research for the Division of Nursing in the federal Bureau of Health Professions (BHP) (Vector Research, 1995), also predicts substantial growth in demand for RNs, although smaller than projected by the BLS. The initial GSDM forecast released in 1991 predicted a 26 percent increase in the number of RNs employed in the United States between 1990 and 2005. This forecast (see Figure 3.2) projects a net increase in the number of employed RNs of 400,000 (U.S. Bureau of Health Professions, 1991).

Institute Of Medicine (IOM) Report. In January 1996 a committee appointed by the IOM issued its report on the future of nursing in hospitals and nursing homes. The report reviewed existing literature and data on the nursing workforce in these settings and received testimony from numerous nurses, nursing

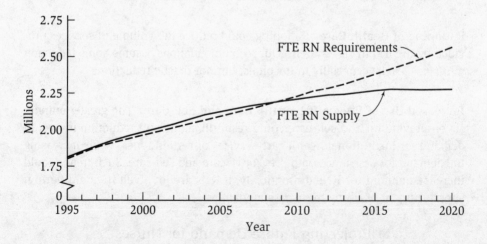

Figure 3.2. Projections of Supply and Requirements for Full-Time Equivalent Registered Nurses as of December 31, 1995–2020.

Source: Wunderlich, Sloan, and Davis, 1996.

organizations, and others involved in health care (Wunderlich, Sloan, and Davis, 1996). The IOM committee concluded that the aggregate supply of RNs is adequate to meet demand at least in the near term, but there may be a need for a higher percentage of RNs educated at the graduate or bachelor's level.

Pew Health Professions Commission. The Pew Health Professions Commission in its third report reached a very different conclusion than the other three reports. Focusing on reductions in hospital beds across the country, the Pew Commission concluded that there would be a major decrease in the demand for nurses. It estimated that there would be a loss of 200,000 to 300,000 RN positions in hospitals nationwide if all excess bed capacity were eliminated (Pew Health Professions Commission, 1995, p. 32). This estimate was derived from analyses of hospital bed capacity that suggest that if all persons in the United States were hospitalized at health maintenance organization (HMO) rates and all hospitals maintained an occupancy rate of 67 percent, there would be an excess of nearly 500,000 hospital beds. Even if average utilization were 50 percent above HMO rates, there would be an excess of over 223,000 beds. Given that most hospitals have a ratio of 1 to 1.25 RNs per hospital bed, closure of these beds would lead to a reduction of roughly 200,000 to 300,000 RN positions if RN-to-bed ratios were held constant. The Pew Commission anticipates that some, but by no means all, RNs displaced from hospitals will locate new jobs in nursing.

Assessing Projections of Future Demand for Nurses

Two factors may have converged to limit the accuracy of projections based on historical experience, such as the BLS and BHP models, at least in the short term. First, the organization and financing of health care have changed dramatically in recent years. Until recently, the health care system was driven by cost-based, fee-for-service reimbursement that created little incentive to health facilities and other providers to limit services and costs. Recent changes have led health facilities to scrutinize all of their costs. Because labor is the largest single cost for most facilities and nursing is often the single largest labor cost, many facilities are reassessing their staffing patterns and especially their use of nursing personnel.

The second factor limiting the accuracy of projections is fluctuating nursing wages, particularly RN wages, relative to wages for other occupations. For many years RN salaries were low relative to those of other nurses and other occupations. In the 1980s the average salary of an RN was only 36 percent above the average salary of an LPN or LVN (Wunderlich, Sloan, and Davis, 1996, p. 75), which created an incentive to hire RNs to perform both RN and LPN or LVN tasks along with clerical and housekeeping functions. As nursing salaries rose relative to those of other nursing and nonnursing personnel in the late 1980s and early 1990s, and as health facilities began to face severe competition and pressure to constrain costs, employers began to rethink their staffing patterns. From 1980 to 1992 RN salaries rose an average of 33 percent (adjusted for inflation), in sharp contrast to wages for most U.S. workers, which either fell or stagnated (p. 75). This has widened the gap between RN wages and those of LPNs and LVNs and unlicensed personnel, leading hospitals to question whether the value added by RNs is sufficiently large to justify the higher labor costs. Some hospitals have determined that it is more cost-effective to use LPNs or LVNs and assistive personnel to perform clerical, housekeeping, and patient care tasks for which RN education is not required. These hospitals now use RNs more selectively to supervise LPNs or LVNs, nurse aides, and other assistive personnel.

Recent information indicates that RN wages have been stagnant from 1992 to 1996. Buerhaus and Staiger (1996, p. 1487), examining RNs in the Current Population Survey data on RNs, found no real wage growth from 1992 to 1994. Early 1996 data show an 11 percent increase in RN wages and a 9.5 percent increase in full-time staff nurse wages from 1992 to 1996 (Moses, 1997a). However, because the Consumer Price Index grew 11 percent over the same period, RNs saw no real wage growth and staff RNs saw real wages fall 1.5 percent. This is similar to the pattern prior to the 1986 nursing shortage, and may be a factor contributing to the lack of growth in workforce participation rates of RNs over the past four years.

The fluctuations in nurse wages, the critical mediating variable between demand and supply, are difficult to track and quantify. And in a period of rapid transition in health care like the mid-1990s, it is even more difficult to project trends and impacts of these important factors. Published forecasts of demand and supply should clarify the time period on which the forecasts are based. Any forecasts based on data prior to 1992 should be examined very carefully because of the major changes in trends that have occurred since then. For similar reasons, forecasts of future demand beyond four or five years should be interpreted with caution.

Assumptions About the Impact on the Nursing Workforce

These changes in the organization and financing of health care are already affecting the nursing workforce. Although it is difficult to predict the extent of the impact, many of the basic trends are apparent:

• The overall percentage of RNs working in hospitals as compared to other settings is expected to continue to drop. As noted in Chapter Two, currently 60 percent of RNs work in hospitals, 6.5 percent less than in 1992. However, the numbers of nurse practitioners (who may substitute for both physicians and registered nurses) and patient care assistants (who will substitute for registered nurses, LPNs and LVNs, and nurse aides for routine tasks) are likely to increase.

• The increased acuity of patients and the need to manage patient care across a variety of institutional settings is likely to create a need for a higher skill mix of nursing personnel in hospitals and nursing homes. This may lead to increased use of nurses with BSNs and advanced training. However, the increase in patient acuity is not expected to fully offset the effects of the decline in hospital utilization on hospital RN employment.

• The growth of ambulatory care settings will increase the demand for nurse practitioners and assistive personnel. However, ambulatory care sites use far fewer staff than hospitals that operate twenty-four hours per day. Thus the anticipated growth in ambulatory care is not expected to generate significant new demand for RNs.

• Home care, which uses RNs extensively, is expected to grow, but because only 7.3 percent of all RN jobs were in home care in 1996 (Moses, 1997b), this will compensate for only a fraction of the losses in hospital-based RN jobs.

• The need for nurses for case management, quality assurance, and utilization review positions is likely to grow in many settings, including managed care plans. However, as with other settings, growth in demand for nurses in such positions will absorb only a fraction of RNs displaced from hospitals.

• Ongoing efforts to reengineer health care services will extend the substitution of lower-paid workers for higher-paid workers wherever possible and reduce staffing requirements in all health care settings, including hospitals, nursing homes, and home care.

Our Demand Projections

The projections that flow from these critical assumptions follow. Separate assessments are made for the major classes of nursing personnel.

The demand for nurse practitioners (NPs) will continue to grow significantly for the foreseeable future. NPs will provide increasingly complex services and care in all settings. As a less expensive option to physicians, NPs will be in demand in acute care settings as direct care givers, patient care managers, and leaders of acute care delivery teams. Precise estimates are difficult to develop, but we envision an increase in demand for NPs of between 50 and 75 percent over the next decade.

The demand for RNs without preparation for advanced practice is expected to decline by about 10 percent over the next ten to fifteen years, due to anticipated significant reductions in the numbers of acute care hospital beds. If not for anticipated increases in acuity of care in hospital settings, job loss would be even greater. One positive outcome is that RNs will be required to do fewer housekeeping and clerical tasks, and as a result may have more time to devote to patient care services as well as supervision of LPNs and LVNs and other support staff. RNs will also increasingly be asked to follow patients across institutional settings. This will be a major change in how RNs currently practice, particularly for RNs educated at the associate and diploma level, who have traditionally been educated to function in the hospital setting.

This assessment is consistent with the observations of Aiken, Sochalski, and Anderson (1996), who suggest that RNs seem to be getting what they have sought for years: for example, higher pay, less menial work, and more management responsibility. If this pattern continues, it could result in greater job satisfaction and longer nursing careers, helping to offset the impact of later entry in practice and general aging of the RN workforce. Conversely, if total nursing staff in hospitals continue to decrease, or the changes previously noted are not perceived as positive by RNs, satisfaction and labor force participation rates may decrease as well.

As NPs and RNs assume roles as leaders of care teams, the demand for patient care technicians, medical assistants, and other multiskilled personnel will continue to grow in both hospital and nonhospital settings. Although there is considerable commonality among these unlicensed personnel across facilities and geographic areas, they are still too new to be able to develop reliable estimates of the current supply, let alone future demand. However, we anticipate significant growth in the demand for unlicensed multiskilled personnel over the next decade, provided they continue to generate cost savings for health care facilities. This growth will likely continue to be associated with comparable declines in demand for other types of workers, including RNs. As the numbers of unlicensed, multiskilled health care workers grow, there may be pressure to license them. This, in turn, would create pressure for higher salaries, which would cause LPNs and LVNs to become more attractive members of health care teams.

How LPNs and LVNs fit into the patterns and trends just described is not clear. The major determining factors will be LPN and LVN salaries and flexibility relative to those of RNs and unlicensed assistive personnel. In most states LPNs and LVNs are permitted to administer medications, which is an advantage over unlicensed assistive personnel. However, if wages of LPNs and LVNs are significantly higher than those of unlicensed assistive personnel, cost-conscious facilities will probably decide to use such personnel.

FACTORS AFFECTING THE FUTURE SUPPLY OF NURSES

Many factors will influence the supply of nurses in the future. Five that are especially important for planners and policymakers are described here.

Responsiveness of Schools of Nursing

Schools of nursing have historically responded relatively quickly to imbalances between supply and demand, in contrast to medical schools. Not only are nursing education programs much shorter than those of medical schools and subsequent residency training programs, they are also not as highly regulated.

Clinical training opportunities for nurses have become more competitive in recent years, especially for primary care programs, as undergraduates compete for fewer hospital placements and graduate students compete with medical students and NP and physician assistant (PA) students for primary care placements. In addition, productivity concerns of managed care organizations have limited use of managed care settings for primary care training. An American Association of Colleges of Nursing (AACN) survey (Mezibov, 1997) reported that 23 percent of the responding nursing programs limited their admissions to their NP programs due to insufficient clinical sites and another 27 percent cited too few faculty.

In the past, schools of nursing have taken advantage of their ability to respond quickly to adjust their production in response to changes in demand. This can be seen graphically in Figure 3.3, which shows trends in graduations from RN, LPN or LVN, and APN programs in the United States. Both associate and baccalaureate programs have been quite flexible, shrinking their graduations by more than 15 percent in the early 1980s and subsequently increasing production substantially in response to shortages of nurses in the late 1980s. There is no reason to believe that nursing schools will lose this flexibility to adjust their

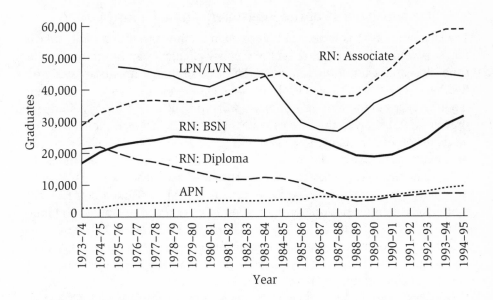

Figure 3.3. Graduations from Nursing Education Programs: RN, APN, and LPN/LVN, 1973–74 to 1994–95.

Source: National League for Nursing, 1996

production to meet the demands of the labor market. In fact, recent enrollment data suggest that schools, or at least potential students, are already responding to publicity about the oversupply of nurses. In 1996, master's degree enrollment decreased by 3.4 percent from 1995, the first decrease since 1988, and baccalaureate enrollments dropped for the second year in a row, with a drop of 6.2 percent from 1995 to 1996 (Berlin, Bednash, and Scott, 1997).

In spite of the flexibility shown by schools of nursing in adjusting enrollments, responses by schools and students who select nursing as a career tend to lag behind market realities because of delays in disseminating employment information. Changes in admissions and enrollments are generally not felt as changes in supply until current students graduate two to four years in the future.

Educational policy lags even further behind the market. The changes occurring in the RN labor market in recent years are only now affecting educational policies and budgets. This creates the risk of a whiplash effect if the new educational policies take effect after the labor market has already adjusted to new conditions. Educational policy should be very carefully formulated to promote long-term goals in the education of nurses, and the potential negative effects on long-term supply should be carefully considered. Perhaps public officials should consider options for improving the timeliness of data collection and reporting so that decisions about educational capacity and enrollment as well as subsidies and incentives can be based on the latest information and insights.

Responsiveness of the Registered Nurse Labor Market

The short-run responsiveness of RNs to changes in wages gives some indication of whether the market, absent any policy changes, can return to equilibrium. Research examining this question has had mixed results. A study by Buerhaus (1991) found that wage levels were not a significant factor for explaining differences in the numbers of hours worked by RNs. However, a study by Brewer (1996) showed that wages were a significant factor in the labor force participation of RNs. Other studies (Link, 1992; Brewer, 1997) have estimated the importance of wages and other factors on RN labor force participation.

In economic terms, most nurses are considered secondary workers because most have spouses who also work. Buerhaus (1995) concluded that RNs are more likely than most workers to respond to changes in personal economic prospects. For example, as income levels of spouses increase, RNs appear to become more willing to reduce their participation in the work force. Depending on the state of the economy, some RNs leave practice when their spouses' income is "comfortably high" (Moses, 1994).

In policy terms, opportunities for influencing nursing wages are limited. It is more important for planners and policymakers to understand the magnitude and speed of response of labor to wage changes than to be able to control wages. Lags in the collection, reporting, and dissemination of wage data delay responses by both nurses and employers. However, if wage levels are not sufficiently effective in influencing appropriate changes in the labor supply over the short run, then policies that influence the long run supply through educational subsidies become relatively more important.

Older Age at Entry into Practice of Nursing

Chapter Two describes the upward trend in nurses' average age at entry to practice that has persisted for over a decade. The IOM committee observed that "if current trends continue, by the year 2000 only about 7 percent will be under 30 years" (Wunderlich, Sloan, and Davis, 1996, p. 73). This means that nurses entering the workforce are likely to work two or three fewer years than their counterparts sixteen years ago. If the trend toward older entry into practice continues, the reduction in the availability of RNs will be even greater. An average decline in workforce participation of three years would represent a 10 percent decrease in average lifetime productivity for new RNs, a very significant long-term effect. There is nothing to suggest that these trends will not continue in the future.

The Aging of the Nursing Workforce

Chapter Two also documents the steady rise in the average age of RNs over the past twenty years. The IOM report suggests that this trend may compromise the ability of RNs to meet the demands of hospital settings, because older RNs may have more difficulty coping with the physical demands of hospital practice (Wunderlich, Sloan, and Davis, 1996, p. 73). It is possible that greater use of patient care assistants and clinical clerks to handle menial tasks will make hospital practice more attractive for RNs. However, there is no reason to suspect that nurses will alter their past patterns of moving out of hospitals as they get older. In fact, the current trend toward more intense nursing care in hospitals may accelerate this "outmigration" in the future.

Alternatives to Nursing

There may be a growing number of opportunities for RNs to work outside nursing, especially in a strong economy. No research has examined RN work histories to determine which nurses are most likely to return to nursing if they are not currently employed, how long RNs are typically out of the workforce for young children, or how likely an RN would be to return to clinical nursing as opposed to other options. Career options for RNs that do not require the RN license but give the RN a comparative advantage, such as managerial positions in health care organizations, may be expanding in the health care marketplace. However, once an RN begins work outside nursing, she or he is unlikely to return to active patient care.

RECOMMENDATIONS FOR SCHOOLS OF NURSING

Based on these projections and considerations, we have several recommendations for nursing education programs:

The recent increase in nurse practitioner graduates appears sufficient to meet the anticipated increases in demand.

The recent expansion of educational capacity should be sufficient in aggregate to meet the expected increase in demand. Therefore, other than expansion to meet specific local or regional needs, we recommend that nursing programs delay further expansion of NP programs for several years. In addition, in the long run, demand for NPs could decline in some specialties and geographic regions if physicians compete directly with NPs for employment, which is a possibility as many observers predict a major surplus of specialist physicians. This recommendation concerns aggregate enrollment, not individuals' career choices. (Because demand is still growing, an NP education is still an excellent choice for an individual RN.)

The number of new RNs should be reduced in aggregate by about 10 percent per year (or approximately 9,300 RNs).

Enrollment and graduation data should be closely monitored. The NLN reported that admissions were down 7.5 percent in 1995, and enrollments had declined 2.7 percent, after beginning to decline in 1994 (Brewer, 1997). Whether this is a deliberate response by nursing programs or the result of a shift in student interest is not clear. However, this moderate response should help to avoid problems of overproduction of RNs as the health care delivery system is redesigned and the health care workforce reengineered over the coming decade.

The number of associate degree and diploma RN programs should decrease and baccalaureate programs should increase.

Consideration should be given to promoting full-time enrollment of generic bachelor's students in order to lower the age of students in nursing. We further recommend that there be greater opportunities for associate- and diploma-educated RNs to obtain baccalaureate degrees. These initiatives will support the greater use of RNs as patient care team managers in inpatient settings for persons with highly acute and complex needs, as well as coordinators and care givers of patients across multiple settings. Increasing opportunities for diploma and associate degree RNs to obtain BSNs will also assist RNs in rural and inner city areas who may have less access to generic (entry-level) BSN programs. We further recommend that hospitals and other employers of RNs become partners in this effort. Federal subsidies for nursing education should be realigned to promote these goals, which are consistent with those of many nursing organizations.

> Educators should carefully monitor future local and national
> workforce trends and be prepared to adjust the size and content of
> their programs quickly to avoid serious imbalances in the future.

The health care system is evolving too rapidly and the workforce marketplace is too dynamic to be able to predict supply and demand beyond two or three years with any certainty. This indicates the need for the systematic collection, analysis, and dissemination of additional data on supply and demand on a regular basis. These data are critical if educators are to make appropriate decisions about the size and content of nursing education programs.

CONCLUSION

Overall demand for RNs will decline over the next ten to fifteen years in the United States, primarily due to reductions in the size of acute inpatient facilities and increased competition among health care professionals. Increased patient acuity in acute care settings and greater opportunities for RNs in ambulatory care and home care settings will generate an increase in demand, but this will not be as large as the decreases due to hospital downsizing. It is probable, however, over the short term, that enrollment will relatively quickly match the decrease in demand because nursing educators and prospective students historically have responded quickly to shifts in demand. In the longer term, there are risks of a nursing shortage. The lags in the response of the labor supply, potential sharp reductions in educational subsidies, and decreased participation by an aging nursing workforce may ultimately reduce the supply of nurses to a level that is inadequate to meet the ultimate increase in demand due to the aging of the population.

References

Aiken, L. H., Sochalski, J., and Anderson, G. F. "Downsizing the Hospital Nursing Workforce." *Health Affairs,* 1996, *15*(4), 88–92.

Berlin, L. E., Bednash, G. D., and Scott, D. L. *1996–1997 Enrollments and Graduations in Baccalaureate and Graduate Programs in Nursing.* Washington, D.C.: American Association of Colleges of Nursing, 1997.

Brewer, C. S. "The Rollercoaster Supply of Registered Nurses: Lessons from the Eighties." *Research in Nursing Health,* 1996, *19*, 345–357.

Brewer, C. S. "Through the Looking Glass: The Labor Market for Nurses in the 21st Century." *Nursing and Health Care,* Sept./Oct. 1997.

Brewer, C. S. "The History and Future of Nursing Labor Research in a Cost Control Environment." *Research in Nursing and Health,* Apr. 1998.

Buerhaus, P. I. "Economic Determinants of Annual Hours Worked by Registered Nurses." *Medical Care,* 1991, *29*(1), 181–195.

Buerhaus, P. I. "Economic Pressures Building in the Hospital Employed RN Labor Market." *Nursing Economics,* 1995, *13,* 137–141.

Buerhaus, P. I., and Staiger, D. O. "Managed Care and the Nurse Labor Market." *Journal of the American Medical Association,* 1996, *276*(18), 1487–1493.

Ferguson, L. Personal communication to author from American Hospital Association, Apr. 9, 1997.

Link, C. "Labor Supply Behavior of Registered Nurses: Female Labor Supply in the Future?" In R. G. Ehrenberg (ed.), *Research in Labor Economics,* 13. Greenwich, Conn.: JAI Press, 1992.

Mezibov, D. (ed.). *AACN Issue Bulletin: A Report on Critical Issues of Concern to Nursing Education and Health Care.* Washington, D.C.: American Association of Colleges of Nursing, Mar. 1997.

Moses, E. B. *The Registered Nurse Population: Findings from the National Sample Survey of Registered Nurses, March 1992.* Rockville, Md.: Division of Nursing, U.S. Bureau of Health Professions, Health Resources and Services Administration, U.S. Department of Health and Human Services, 1994.

Moses, E. B. "Advance Notes II from the National Sample Survey of Registered Nurses, March 1996." [http://www.hrsa.dhhs.gov/bhpr/dn/advnotel.htm] Rockville, Md.: Division of Nursing, U.S. Bureau of Health Professions, 1997a.

Moses, E. B. *The Registered Nurse Population: Findings from the National Sample Survey of Registered Nurses, March 1996.* Rockville, Md.: Division of Nursing, U.S. Bureau of Health Professions, Health Resources and Services Administration, U.S. Department of Health and Human Services, 1997b.

National League for Nursing. *Nursing Datasource.* New York: National League for Nursing, 1996.

Pew Health Professions Commission. *Critical Challenges: Revitalizing the Health Professions for the Twenty-First Century.* San Francisco: UCSF Center for the Health Professions, 1995.

Spetz, J. *Hospital Staffing of Nurses in California from 1977 to 1994.* San Francisco: Public Policy Institute of California, Aug. 1996.

U.S. Bureau of Health Professions. *Eighth Report to the President and Congress on the Status of Health Personnel in the United States.* U.S. Bureau of Health Professions, Health Resources and Services Administration, Public Health Service, U.S. Department of Health and Human Services, 1991.

U.S. Bureau of Labor Statistics. *Monthly Labor Review,* 1995, *118*(11).

Vector Research, Inc. *General Services Demand Model: Executive Review Document.* Ann Arbor, Mich.: Vector Research, Inc., May 1995.

Wunderlich, G. S., Sloan, F. A., and Davis, C. K. (eds.). *Nursing Staff in Hospitals and Nursing Homes: Is It Adequate?* Washington, D.C.: National Academy Press, 1996.

PART TWO

THE CHANGING NATURE OF NURSES' WORK

Demand for Nurses in
Specific Employment Settings

CHAPTER FOUR

The Impact of Managed Care and Integrated Delivery Systems on Registered Nurse Education and Practice

Barbara Balik

With this chapter, the book moves from consideration of the number of RNs needed in the future to the skills and competencies that will be demanded of them in the emerging managed care–oriented environment. Balik describes the evolution of systems of managed care from cost avoidance to value improvement to health improvement. In each stage the role and function of the RN will change considerably, but will draw heavily on the developmental and psychosocial strengths that have become so integral to nursing professionalism. Although these elements are already a part of the nursing curriculum, the author suggests ways to focus and improve on this orientation.

The evolution of health care systems and the emergence of the market metaphor described in Chapter One are affecting future nursing roles and responsibilities. Understanding the current state of health care and expected trends equips nursing leaders to anticipate possible future contexts for practice and informs their work in advancing patient care systems. The purpose of this chapter is to describe one model of evolution of managed care and integrated care delivery systems. Within the model, the chapter offers nursing leaders' assessments of the impact of the managed care evolution on the role and scope of nursing in the emerging systems. It also includes suggestions for potential competencies for nursing professionals and leaders as well as examples of practice and organizational changes. The review also challenges thinking about education and encourages ongoing discourse among leaders regarding nursing education, practice, licensure, and multidisciplinary learning. The model moves toward interdisciplinary perspectives in both practice and education based on client need and required practitioner competencies.

Literature is limited to support the exploration of nursing in the evolving environment. The insight and talent of skillful leaders who formed a expert panel are reflected here. They draw from experiences in health care systems in California,

New Mexico, Massachusetts, and Minnesota. Their thoughtfulness and innovation on the leading edge of health care is inspiring and illuminating.

ASSUMPTIONS ABOUT THE FUTURE OF MANAGED CARE AND INTEGRATED CARE DELIVERY SYSTEMS

Projections of future demand for and scope of practice of any health care provider depend on the assumptions made regarding the future health care system and the population it will serve. This chapter is grounded in assumptions about the future of health care in the United States consistent with those outlined in Chapter One. Additional assumptions concern the emergence of a chronic condition/health model for delivery of health care services and a shift in delivery systems' focus from individual to community needs.

As life expectancy increases and the "baby boom" generation reaches retirement, the number of persons living with chronic conditions will increase dramatically. This trend will further stretch the current acute care/cure oriented system, leading to its deconstruction and transformation into a chronic condition/health oriented system. Establishment of a chronic condition/health model will be accompanied by a transition in care delivery systems' objectives from management of costs to genuine management of care. This shift requires recognition that health care providers currently lack the professional and educational framework to serve the public's changing health care needs. The skills of interdependency required to achieve a chronic condition/health model of services constitute a significant gap in meeting these needs. Interdependency includes recognition of the patient or consumer as partner in the design and delivery of services.

This chapter also envisions that care delivery systems will not continue to focus narrowly on the medical needs of individual enrollees, but will instead expand systems' missions and activities to address the health of the communities in which enrollees reside. The pressure on health care delivery systems to respond to community needs will intensify due to the growing recognition that health status is not solely dependent on access to medical technology or sufficient numbers of providers but also on socioeconomic factors (such as education, safety, nutrition), behavioral choices (such as smoking, nutrition, seat belt use), and access to health-promoting interventions rather than later attempts at restoration. The line between social and clinical needs is being redrawn. Effective response to these community needs requires greater partnership between health care organizations and public and social agencies to meet demographic changes. However, care delivery systems' efforts to address community health are rather limited at present. To date no integrated delivery system in the United

States has demonstrated a significant improvement in community health as a result of its integration.

Given the assumptions, discussion of the specific topic of the impact of managed care and integrated care delivery systems on the demand for nursing practitioners begins with a description of current reality. The literature shows a country and communities seeking to make meaning of the current and projected environment (a list of important articles appears at the end of this chapter). Lack of a common language and clarity regarding the desired future results in confusion. The lack of common language is reflected in the array of definitions of managed care and integrated systems developed to achieve managed care (Hicks, Stallmeyer, and Coleman, 1992; Madison and Konrad, 1988; United HealthCare Corporation, 1994; Halvorsen, 1993). The confusion leads to disarray, yet paradoxically also provides opportunity for innovation and radical improvement of a system in distress. The model described here reflects aspects of all the definitions with an emphasis on the ultimate public accountability to promote health rather than solely intervene to treat illness.

IMPACT OF MANAGED CARE AND INTEGRATED CARE DELIVERY SYSTEMS ON PROVIDERS

Goldsmith, Goran, and Nackel (1995, p. 18) anticipate that "as the market matures, managed care enterprises will be driven to fundamentally redefine their business. Managed care firms will follow a predictable path of redefinition of their business as growth plateaus and traditional strategies for generating earnings no longer yield measurable gain." They predict a three-stage evolution, from event-driven cost avoidance to value improvement and finally to health improvement. The evolution addresses the concern raised by Mila Aroskar (1995, p. 83) and other ethicists that the language of managed care is only a euphemism for turning medical care decisions into business decisions. The three phases illustrate development toward a health improvement model that moves beyond solely medical or business decisions to an integrated view of health.

This framework also calls attention to the adaptive challenges facing health professionals. Heifetz (1994) stated that the work of leaders in a complex world is the identification of adaptive challenges, not technical fixes. Heifetz describes adaptive work as the learning required to address conflicts in the values people hold or to decrease the gap between the values people stand for and the reality they face. Adaptive work thus requires a change of those involved in their values, beliefs, or behavior (p. 22). The adaptive challenge in health care services and systems are found in the second and third stages—value improvement and health improvement.

Cost Avoidance Stage

Managed care systems in the United States are at varied stages of maturity. The cost avoidance stage results in the most dramatic short-term shift in the need for types of providers, most particularly specialty physicians and acute care nurses. The consequences of this shift are reflected in the current RN employment patterns described in Chapter Two and the short-term projections of future demand for RNs reviewed in Chapter Three.

However, local decisions about provider requirements cannot be based on aggregate data. Health care needs and the systems through which they are met vary widely among communities. The services and providers needed in tribal lands in northern Minnesota are very different from those required in inner-city Detroit. Thus appropriate responses in individual communities depend on local requirements and the current and future adequacy of supplies of required providers.

The work in the cost avoidance stage of managed care is exemplified by activities best described as "fiddling with the edges." The efforts rework the acute care/illness model to maintain the current system. Health care organizations strive to maintain the financial picture of the past, the revenue stream, the boundaries of authority, power, and professional disciplines, and the limited role of the consumer. Costs are managed through restrictions, oversight, double checks, provider discounting, and reviews following service delivery.

A variety of actions appear: reengineering, hospital consolidations and eventual closures, and the development of new service ventures to capture market share. Partnerships between physicians, hospitals, clinics, health plans, and former competitors are prevalent. Use of providers other than physicians to meet primary care needs begins or expands. Quality improvement efforts start to examine core systems particularly in the acute care settings. As leaders in this phase take the risk of honestly examining the current system, the difficulties of changing such a complex enterprise surface.

Fiddling with the edges results in activities but few changes in the nature and function of the health care system. Often absent is a rethinking of the acute care model and development of a health system model. Building ambulatory sites and extending clinic hours do not transform the mindset of the nature of the services and the continuum involved. Moving from the event-driven cost avoidance stage of managed care requires rethinking health care delivery services.

Value Improvement Stage

The second stage of value improvement begins to surface the need for service transformation, or the adaptive challenges, rather than solely merger or rearrangement. Acute care becomes part of a larger system of care rather than its center and represents a serious drain on the finances of health care delivery systems, particularly because it requires increased capital investment. Public health models that are based on concepts of prevention acknowledge chronic conditions as drivers of needs emerge. A generally healthy aging population that develops chronic conditions demands different services. Nursing and other professional disciplines integrate into the whole and grapple with the interdependencies required in the changing system. This stage requires an examination of the processes of services, the interdependencies of family and providers, the questioning of contribution of providers and interventions to overall outcomes and value to the consumer (the user of the services) and customer (purchaser of the services), and redesign of the system of services as opposed to solely looking toward improvement of services.

Health care delivery leaders begin to recognize that significant changes in the system are the only way to control costs and improve the overall delivery process. This recognition results in broader redesign efforts paired with Total Quality Improvement activities; clinical guidelines that address all providers and the full continuum of health and illness; the evolution of care management and health risk assessment; a focus on appropriateness and functional outcomes; and a close examination of types of services (surgical interventions, drugs, laboratory tests, specialists) and their contribution to outcomes. Leaders face the challenges of more informed customers, such as businesses, who demand that providers demonstrate effective and responsible use of resources to maximize efficiency in delivery of services as well as the speed with which employees return to work and family functions.

This stage challenges professionals and the established historical boundaries of roles and practice sites. The deconstruction of historical hierarchies and domains of practice begin. Examples include the emergence of the primary care physician rather than specialist as the focal point of medical services and challenges to the assumption that only physicians can deliver the bulk of primary care services. The need for RNs in acute care settings stabilizes as this phase of redesign is completed and surplus hospital capacity diminishes. These examples represent the beginning of dramatic shifts in the established structure of health care.

Health Improvement Stage

The third stage, health improvement, focuses on population-based health status improvement and is both old and new. Public health concepts, marginalized in the high-tech acute care environment, are now emerging as the next evolution of managed care. Seen as the key to truly improving health and reducing health service costs, this stage links historical public health models with pooled risk capitation, prediction and targeted case management, and identification of community and environmental factors. It requires multidisciplinary teams whose skills move beyond the traditional health services delivery arena to epidemiology and technological skills that support health improvement. This stage also demands more from the consumer and customer. Achievement of health improvement depends on the long-term adaptive changes required to have an impact on health status indicators.

Few examples of this stage of evolution exist. The Healthy Communities efforts provide a model for potential impact on provider skills and location of practice. Healthy Communities is a national effort supported by the Healthcare Forum, W. K. Kellogg Foundation, Healthier Communities Partnership, and a variety of other health care and community organizations. Their commitment is to work in partnership in communities to address a broad range of services and needs identified by community members as important to health. Healthy Communities concepts focus on communities, not individuals, and the partnerships search for a framework that will help redefine the way health is achieved in this country. The search is for understanding and efforts that will promote new strategies leading toward the creation of health in communities rather than strategies that merely improve the approaches to treating illness.

This effort to move upstream, toward prevention, is grounded in the recognition that most health conditions are not caused by lack of access to medical technology or insufficient numbers of providers but rather are associated with socioeconomic factors, such as employment, education, safety; behavioral choices, such as smoking, seat belt use, nutrition; and access to preventive or health-promoting interventions rather than treatment after conditions have developed. Healthy Communities activities are examples of community leaders, including health care leaders, addressing collaboratively the relationships between health and such key components of living and working environments as education, employment, crime, and spiritual well-being. The recognition is that no one sector can sufficiently address the interconnected factors involved in developing health in communities. The concepts stem from the belief that there are insufficient resources to continue the downstream intervention, after illness or complications develop—a belief that challenges the foundation of the present health care system.

This perspective is consistent with the public's views about community health. A telephone survey of Americans commissioned by the Healthcare Forum in 1994 for its study *What Creates Health?* listed determinants of a healthy community. The participants listed low crime rate, a good place to bring up children, good schools, high environmental quality, and good jobs as major determinants.

Allina Health System actively participates in a number of Healthy Communities partnerships. Two examples are the West Seventh Partnership in St. Paul, whose efforts are focused on youth programs and employment efforts; and the Violence Prevention Partnership, whose commitment is to specific, neighborhood efforts to improve safe environments, early identification of violence in households, and mobilization of residents and providers toward a safe community.

ROLES AND SCOPE FOR NURSING IN EMERGING SYSTEMS

The impact of value improvement and health improvement stages in managed care systems on nursing providers are linked and reflect a continuum of changes. The expert panel identified several major challenges to adaptation of RNs' roles and scope of practice to meet the needs of emerging systems.

One major challenge is the need to match patient-client needs to the level of nursing competency rather than solely focus on educational credentials and licensure to determine nurses' progression from one role to another. Reliance on credentials and licensure as the sole determinants of health care provider competency without demonstration of contribution to consumer outcome is a limited path for viewing the future of nursing or any other health care provider.

A second challenge concerns assessment of the number of clinicians needed and their distribution based on demographics, epidemiological descriptors, and health status indicators across all settings, but particularly in community-based settings within a geographical community. The need for clinicians requires assessment on a community, state, and national level in order to examine all levels of the health care system, to identify causes of shortages and surpluses, and to develop public policy to address a variety of needs.

The integration of technology as a platform for practice rather than an adjunct constitutes a third challenge. Basic computer skills, telecare, phone triage, decision support protocols, and common data sets begin to remove the historical boundaries of care settings and on ownership of data. Information systems also function as decision-making tools that are foundational to current and future practice.

A fourth set of challenges encompasses the current definition of cognitive and other skills required for practice. Immediate skills required in the emerging integrated care delivery systems include the following:

- Competencies to practice in a variety of peer unobserved settings with little direct supervision and the ability to consult through remote or technologically linked resources
- Integration of care across settings and with other providers
- Development of qualitative and quantitative skills needed to integrate quality, measurement, outcomes assessment, and research into the scope of practice
- Telephone care management
- Use, development, and systematic evaluation of care protocols

The specific mix of skills required of RNs varies somewhat among settings. Rural community case management is heavily reliant on telephone and remote computer linkages. Management of complex and chronically ill populations such as those with diabetes or congestive heart failure requires strong skills in physical assessment and patient teaching. Health plans seek nurses who can complete risk assessments for new health plan enrollees and use care protocols to ensure that individuals receive appropriate, cost-effective interventions to maximize health. Specific examples in the Allina system follow.

The Family Beginnings Program is a partnership between the Allina health plan, Medica, and the United Hospital Birth Center. Developed to assist women who choose a shorter inpatient postpartum stay, the program focuses on total pregnancy health and preparation in partnership with the family and the obstetrical provider. Services include phone assessment, mailing of appropriate educational material after the assessment, phone contact each trimester, and follow-up after discharge. Registered nurses are the primary providers. Nurse time averages one hour per client. Preliminary results show higher prenatal class attendance, lower preterm birth rates, and a higher breast feeding success rate.

Allina has also developed new roles for nurses in delivering care to persons at the opposite end of the lifespan. Medica leaders in the Center for Healthy Aging were concerned about the at-risk seniors enrolled through a new health plan product. Without a means of managing the moderate- and high-risk population, the cost trend for this group would exceed appropriate levels. Advanced practice nurses in the acute care settings identified the ability to offer short-term case management in conjunction with home care providers to prevent hospitalizations, shorten nursing home stays, and reduce overall utilization of resources.

All Allina acute care redesign efforts have concentrated on maximizing RN time as coordinator and integrator of care with a multidisciplinary emphasis. Team environments are integral to all care settings and bring the strengths of all disciplines together to maximize patient care outcomes. There is less emphasis on nonnursing tasks and more discussion of what the work is, why it is done, who can do it, who should do it, and how it can most effectively be done. The overemphasis on nonnursing tasks in the past has led to compartmentalization of patient care with an abundance of single-role participants. Clarity about the nature of the work and why it is done in the first place also results in assessing the drivers of patient care resources and nursing practice in acute care settings. Although time spent on activities not requiring professional background is important to assess, the significant driver of nursing practice and nursing resources is often physician practice patterns and communication among disciplines. All major drivers of nursing resources must be evaluated. Failure to address the system as a whole will limit the long-term success of redesign efforts. This expanded view of redesign of services is consistent with a value improvement stage of evolution.

In the outpatient setting, Allina emphasizes team practice with major roles for advance practice nurses (APNs). Allina has historically referred to "providers" in the clinics. This inclusive term applies to physicians, nurse practitioners, physician assistants, and all other professional care givers. There is a consistent need for advanced practice nurses (APNs) in primary care outpatient settings. The model of APN as coordinator and team provider for complex conditions such as diabetes, neurological conditions, and congestive heart failure is rapidly growing. The intent is to keep the population as a whole healthier and diminish hospitalizations.

Allina and other integrated delivery systems support the collaboration between physicians and APN through a focus on clinical outcomes, collegial relationships, an expectation of multidisciplinary work, and alignment of incentives. Physicians' responses to APNs in Allina range from enthusiastic support to skepticism. The single largest barrier is alignment of incentives, especially financial. Physicians are most threatened when other providers (APNs, pharmacists, other physicians) impinge on their practice scope, patient relationships, future patient population base, or income. The tension between provider groups will continue until rationalized incentives focus on population health outcomes or other measures that diminish the individualized perspective and advances the interdependent model of care.

Allina has two major approaches to changing the system of care. The first, the clinical care model (see Figure 4.1), develops a multidisciplinary description of best of practice in care; the second is participation in the Institute for Healthcare Improvement Breakthrough Series and Project IMPROVE. Advanced practice nurses are essential members of the best-of-practice design groups and the clinical action or implementation groups. The breakthrough groups bring together groups of health care organizations that share a commitment to making major, rapid changes that lead to breakthrough improvement: lower cost and better outcomes at the same time. Each breakthrough collaborative lasts approximately one year, includes thirty to forty organizations, focuses on a single topic area, and concentrates on learning the best scientific and process knowledge available and putting that knowledge into practice for rapid improvement. Allina is participating in four breakthrough groups—reduction of cesarean birth rates, reduction of adverse drug events, improving care and reducing costs in adult intensive care, and open heart surgery. Embedded in both approaches to care system changes is a multidisciplinary focus with visible and essential leadership from nurses.

The work of both initiatives takes care redesign concepts to the next level of sophistication. The system changes demand the assessment of nursing practice patterns, drivers of utilization of nursing services, and sources of nursing

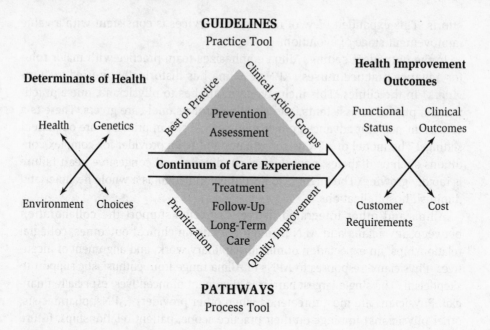

Figure 4.1. Allina Clinical Care Model.

practice variation. These are the major quality and cost issues and move beyond the basic assessment of nursing and nonnursing functions.

Allina acute care hospitals place a heavy emphasis on the competencies required in emerging systems. These competencies include clarity regarding the essence of caring, critical thinking, cross-boundary and multidisciplinary perspectives, coordination and facilitation of care process, direct communication, conflict resolution, awareness of managed care environments, team skills, patient-centered focus, community-based focus or belief that the patient and family begin and end in the community, and eagerness to learn. Redesign of services in all of seventeen Allina acute care facilities identified these skills as essential for success.

Nurses are remarkable in their capacity to build on current strengths and add these additional competencies if they do not have them. The emphasis at Allina is on learning, growth, and choice. Most Allina nurses chose the new and redesigned acute care settings. Some chose different practice settings because these competencies were not consistent with their preferred practice and found other successful practice settings.

Allina uses competency-based tools developed by leaders and staff to reflect the key skills. Assessment includes professional as well as technical proficiency, commitments to caring, team skills and communication capabilities, and the ability to advance the plan of care to the expected outcome. Education offered across Allina includes content on the business of health care, communication and conflict in the workplace, care coordination, and other identified areas of need beyond the advances in care interventions.

Bachelor's degrees are preferred because the curriculums of bachelor of nursing programs in Minnesota teach and develop many of the needed skills. The percentage of bachelor's prepared nurses is gradually increasing in all roles. This is not to say that associate degree prepared nurses are not hired. Their supply and skill make them an available pool of employees. The focus in Allina is on continual learning with tuition assistance, supportive scheduling practices for students, and community-based programs to facilitate progression toward bachelor's degrees. Support and recognition for certification is an additional tool for quality validated in practice and supported by the continued efforts required to maintain certification. An increase in the number of APN positions reflects the need for these practitioners in complex settings. The positions are in primary care, acute care, and continuum-spanning roles.

EDUCATIONAL AND LICENSURE IMPLICATIONS

The evolution of integrated health systems requires a contemporary model for education focused on health improvement. Carol Lindeman (1995) has identified core changes required in nursing education to meet future needs. The expert panel concurred with and expanded on concepts described by Lindeman. The changes the panel suggest represent the seed of the shift in thinking nurses need to function and lead in the evolving environment. They provide a contemporary model for education.

Model Changes

From a provider-identified needs-driven model to an integrated resource-driven model. Learning that every need requires intervention has led to a provider-centered approach to care often accompanied by wide practice variability. It also led to discipline-specific languages and systems that resulted in barriers to integration of services. This lack of integration had led to unnecessary duplication, confusion, and lack of coordination, all of which pose serious obstacles to improving consumers' health and well-being. Health professional- and needs-driven models also reinforced a reductionistic, linear, problem-solving approach rather than an integrative view.

From individual autonomous functioning to interdisciplinary models. Individualistic views limit an outcomes focus and emphasize turf over client improvement.

From episodic to care over the continuum. The change in perspective requires understanding phenomena over time, incorporation of a holistic view, movement away from sole reliance on medical diagnosis, and cognizance of a variety of environmental and relational influences on the determinants of health.

From provider centered to partnership with consumers. The chronic condition/health model can only succeed if consumers are knowledgeable partners in ensuring their health.

From technology as optional tool to technology as foundation of practice. This requires that practice sites advance dramatically in the technology available to support practice, not just to deliver service. The potential for change diminishes when providers are saddled with nineteenth-century information systems.

Core Outcomes

In addition to the new model for education, Lindeman identified core outcomes for nursing education. She described these as outcomes for undergraduate nursing education. However, these competencies can be achieved and sustained in multiple ways and are not solely attained through completion of a specific curriculum or level of education. The basic skills are the following:

- *Critical thinking:* to analyze arguments, construct meaning, view knowledge as a context and as a guide not a rule, and critically reflect on one's own acts and thinking. Of all the competencies discussed, the expert panel highlighted critical thinking as the most foundational and crucial.

- *Relationship skills:* as a mechanism in which health and healing occurs.

- *Care management skills:* different from care provider skills, these skills facilitate the furnishing of the right intervention at the right time, in the right setting, and at the appropriate cost; the ability to look at services as a constellation of care as well as a continuum.

- *Primary care skills:* a health-focused rather than a disease-oriented approach.

- *Community-focused skills:* a community asset focus—the ability to work with community groups and to recognize and tap the power in communities; avoidance of sole reliance on institutions for function.

Additional skills not mentioned by Lindeman but integral to maintaining the others are systems thinking and leadership development. Nurses are excellent systems thinkers as it applies to the health care needs of individuals served. They need to broaden those skills so they can consistently see family and community as part of the system as well as the interrelationships of an array of political, social, and economic variables present when exploring the health of a community.

Discussions with colleagues across the country suggest the gap varies between the vision for education and the current reality. Many educational programs are led by creative, externally oriented deans and faculty in partnership with practice leaders. Talented students emerge equipped with many of the skills needed in all levels of practice. The graduates carry a worldview of constant growth and change and the confidence to build on today's knowledge to meet the future. However, other educational and practice relationships are less effective. Faculty demonstrate little awareness of managed care or the opportunities for influence by nursing. Students emerge much as they have in the past and then grapple with confusion and frustration in a dramatically different practice world. It is as if they had been misled and someone changed the rules.

Leadership and Leadership Development

The ability of integrated delivery systems to integrate patient-client care services across delivery settings and the decision making required to lead services in new systems depend on the stage of evolution. Executives in immature systems may fail to identify, hear, or heed the voice of providers and clinical operations leaders in shaping the systems. The failure comes from both the health care business leaders who think they know how to shape the future and from clinical providers and leaders who guard the status quo and disregard the skills needed to lead organizations. It is a marriage of dismissal and resistance that eventually diminishes both groups. As systems mature in the managed care evolution, partnerships among leaders with a variety of skills and backgrounds, including clinical, emerge to address the demands of future stages. Intimate knowledge of the nature of clinical care is a resource to be tapped and valued when the clinical leaders are willing to shape and create new systems.

The members of the expert panel both identify and exemplify the competencies required: cross-boundary relationships, an abundance mentality to see possibilities, facilitation of diverse groups, reflective practice or the ability to assess their individual behavior and learn from their actions, engagement in dialogue for creation of common meaning, recognition of the heart of the business as care and development of a practice community of service. Strong nursing leadership is essential to successful transformation of health care delivery systems. Developing these transformational leadership skills requires a new approach to learning leadership.

Leadership development is found in most baccalaureate programs and broadened in some master of nursing programs. Learning leadership historically has involved working with an RN in an acute care management role to view positional leadership. Innovative educational programs in schools and continuing education settings are expanding the horizon to the depth and breadth of concepts of shared leadership in all practice roles and settings. This broader context of service needs to be incorporated in all leadership curricula.

Currently, associate degree programs are able to focus on interdependency, reflection in practice, and cross-boundary work. Baccalaureate and master's level programs, with longer student contact, build on the basic competencies to expand the potential of skillful functioning in practice leadership. A variety of learning settings may be used to expand leadership skills. Reflecting on life experiences, reading a wide range of literature, and conferences for personal growth are a sample of learning opportunities in addition to traditional educational programs.

Educational Levels

The debate about nursing educational levels and the distinctions within them has clouded the focus on competency development required by a changing environment. Case management skills are an example of the competencies that are not exclusive to any one educational level. The perspective of some leaders is that case management can only be successfully done by APNs. Yet the changing environment requires a variety of activities within the case management continuum. Basic care coordination that every patient should expect is central to the nursing process and is a competency expected of all RNs. However, resource management and care for a complex population is more appropriate for APN education. Resource management includes planning care that maximizes the client's health in a community-based setting whenever possible with the least resources needed to achieve positive outcomes. One Allina APN leads a congestive heart failure service. Her client base is a population of people who fit at-risk criteria. The care efforts are to enhance care at home and in clinic settings while avoiding hospitalizations. Her practice uses the resources needed to maintain clients' health in the community while avoiding expensive hospitalizations.

Clarity with language and definitions can avoid positional perspectives and lead to informed conversations about the nature and scope of the services practitioners provide and their impact on client outcome. The language used often confuses the conversation and is a barrier to creating common meaning. The confusion then leads to debates about what different levels of preparation mean, what can be learned in practice settings, and who gets to decide. The skills identified in the emerging managed care environment call for well-developed critical, reflective, and analytical thinking, public health practice exposure and framework, and the capacity for broad thinking grounded in the needs of clients in the context of their community. Currently, associate degree education can offer the beginning-level skills in the limited amount of time available for education. Individuals who are continually learning can refine these skills without benefit of educational programs through maximizing their practice and life experience. The current dilemma is how we describe and assess the competencies needed to offer to the public a skillful provider. Until those in service and education develop the new vocabu-

lary of expertise and a means of ensuring expert practice in a changing environment, educational preparation and certification will be the proxy measure.

The value of learning must be held foremost, not how the learning occurs.
Nor should we discount the gains of formal education. The new worldview for
professional development requires embracing a variety of approaches to learning as well as honoring current successful models. The creation of common
meaning and language to better serve the public is the challenge in this complex conversation.

While honoring the broad-based liberal arts tradition of my own academic
development, the challenge is to engage in the discourse about the educational
and practice attributes that support the development of critical, reflective, and
analytical thinkers who demonstrate a capacity for broad perspectives. Reducing the discourse to an assumption that a bachelor's preparation will develop
those capacities is inaccurate. Although the bachelor's preparation may provide
the best potential for those capacities now, it is too random in its outcome for
reliance on this single approach. The cause and effect dimensions of our current common wisdom related to the bachelor's degree and practice competency
in its broadest definition is too simplistic.

The conversation is often limited to positional perspectives: either the bachelor's degree is the only approach or it is not of value. A true dialogue is warranted to surface the assumptions and beliefs embedded in our positions about
educational preparation and to develop other perspectives than the polar oppo-
sites often found. The dialogue needed addresses the interdependency of educational levels based on competencies, not structure. Advancement of nursing
education and practice will come when we can honestly challenge closely held
assumptions, hold a mirror to each other's perspectives, and create a greater
sense of common meaning. The current shorthand of understanding based on
educational levels and well-entrenched arguments limits us all.

Multidisciplinary Learning

If the philosophy of education and core skills are revitalized in the manner recommended, then advancement in health care may not follow discipline-specific
tracks. Basic education may provide a foundation for further study and practice
in other arenas within the same discipline or in others. The philosophy and
skills described pertain to many providers. The blurring of distinctions can perhaps better serve a changing population whose needs transcend the current
descriptions of nurse, social worker, primary care physician, pharmacist, physical therapist, and the like. The current professional distinction may not match
the community needs and may support discipline interests rather than those of
patients-clients. The foundational skills of an RN may lead to the addition of
competencies as a nurse practitioner or other provider skills traditionally
thought of as those of another discipline, such as social work. The reverse could

also result. The key question asked should be, What professional roles are needed to serve communities and the nation?

This perspective prompts further questions about the desirability of continuing to educate social workers, nurses, physicians, pharmacists, and dieticians separately with distinct practice domains. All health professions share a common need for curriculum in the basic sciences, health care policy, leadership, communication, and cross-boundary practice. Are they the same discipline with varied practice elements? How can we examine the core of what we share and honor the differences that emerge based on distinct service needs? Education and practice settings should focus on defining the skills needed and design education to meet the emerging needs rather than revising the existing systems. "Fiddling around the edges" will not offer long-term success for major systems changes.

If we rethink educational philosophy and core skills expected then licensure requirements follow. Examination of what licensure supports and inhibits is under way in many arenas (Finocchio and others, 1995; Minnesota Organization of Leaders in Nursing, 1996). The issue can be framed as one of competency-based practice rather than licensure. The authors of the report *Reforming Health Care Workforce Regulation* (Finocchio and others 1995, p. vii) conclude that the regulation of the health care workforce will best serve the public's interest by doing the following:

- Promoting effective health outcomes and protecting the public from harm

- Holding regulatory bodies accountable to the public

- Respecting consumers as partners and their right to choose their health care providers from a range of safe options

- Encouraging a flexible, rational, and cost-effective health care system that allows effective working relationships among health care providers

- Facilitating professional and geographic mobility of competent providers.

Leadership in Anticipation of Changes

The drivers of changes discussed in this chapter are managed care and the development of integrated delivery systems. The cause and effect framing may create the impression that the external environment is the only trigger for advancement of nursing practice and related competencies. This conclusion would be misleading as well as inaccurate. Evolution and movement toward health improvement is found in a wide range of communities. The competencies required by the public and changing health care needs do not vary by health care financing. Financing modifications merely accelerate the pressure for change.

The perspectives required by senior nursing leaders to improve nursing practice, whether external pressures are present or not, include the following:

The recognition that articulation of nursing practice competency, changes in education, and other concepts in this chapter are not dependent on managed care. They are concepts that focus on the needs and health of the community served. Leaders can choose to focus on future needs rather than wait for the external forces that may appear.

A commitment to informed practice. Informed caring is the core of nursing practice. Nursing leaders model the commitment to informed caring by asking about qualitative and quantitative data that shapes and improves practice. Leaders also ensure systems are present to provide the data and that practitioners learn how to incorporate data into practice.

An organic rather than mechanistic view of organizational systems. The transitions required are not accomplished by the mechanical approaches of moving boxes in organizations or task lists around. Transitions are founded on the organic and growth-filled belief in system changes.

Intellectual curiosity and a spirit of inquiry, constant challenges to closely held beliefs, and creation of an environment of learning to inform the work and stimulate questions in the act of caring. The grounding in quality improvement principles and tools and organic redesign combined with the freedom to risk provides a nurturing and constantly learning care setting.

"Competition is useless": a commitment to collaboration, not competition. Leaders who will not encourage or accept competition between disciplines, departments, roles, or organizations will advance nursing practice and patient care. The Twin Cities carry a long history as one of the most competitive markets in health care, but the nursing leadership there is one of the most collaborative. The common belief is that advancement of care can only benefit the community as a whole. Colleagues routinely call each other to explore how to grapple with a variety of care and nursing practice issues.

A willingness to share the stories that reflect the environment desired. Stories of care and improvements in services propel individuals and organizations forward. Leaders who are skillful storytellers accelerate transformations.

Creating structures and systems that support the essence of the changes desired. Collaborative decision making thrives in structures that facilitate it. Systems of leadership development foster leaders who embrace informed caring and shared decision making.

Knowledge of true organizational costs. Lack of this knowledge often leads to the view of employees as commodities rather than valued resources. The cost avoidance stage of managed care often results in slash and burn approaches to cost reduction. The experiences of those in more mature markets indicate that this is not a long-term, sustainable approach to cost reduction.

CONCLUSION

The growth of managed care and the formation of integrated care delivery systems stimulate a broader discussion regarding the demand for nurses. Four major themes shape thinking about the demand for nurses in the emerging systems.

The model of health care is shifting.

Client- and family-centered partnerships reshape health care to an emphasis on health improvement and management of chronic conditions. A shift to a model of care based in health across the continuum and on collaboration and interdependency requires a wide range of partnerships. Meeting environmental demands of high quality and controlled costs requires shifting models and partnerships.

Implementation of the new model changes demand for nurses across practice settings and the competencies required for practice.

An increasing demand for RNs continues in home care, subacute care, health plans, and ambulatory settings. The demand is not as large as the reduction in demand in acute care. An increased and accelerating demand for advanced practice nurses exists, especially for those who provide primary care, work with chronic health conditions, or practice in underserved areas. There is an increase in the care coordination capabilities expected for nurses in the acute care setting that may increase the split between nurses who develop those skills in their basic program (currently RNs with baccalaureate degrees) and those who do not (those with associate degrees). Margaret Newman (1990) describes a potential model based on the complexity of patient needs and their linkage to educational preparation or competencies of the RN.

The emphasis on the requirements for nurses may vary with local circumstances.

Differences in demand for RNs across communities are driven by the stage of managed care evolution, local demographics, and local needs. This urges a community-based assessment of the number and type of nursing practitioners. The possibility exists for nursing leaders to advance evolution of nursing practice in service to their communities before the managed care evolution occurs.

Communities or regions need a framework for assessment of current and future nursing practitioner needs. The framework integrates local data regarding current providers (such as number, age, practice site, current skills, gaps in services), community health needs and goals, resources currently in place, particular social supports, and stage of managed care evolution. The assessment from the framework determines a plan for meeting regional needs that shape competencies from current or future practitioners. The framework assists national public policy development, especially in the area of financial support for provider education. Communities or regions are then accountable for identifying and responding to their needs.

The current and anticipated shifts demand changes in education and licensure.

Nursing leaders must articulate an emphasis on competencies demonstrated to facilitate the creation and implementation of a chronic condition/health model based on communities' needs. This model stems from discourse between education and practice communities regarding assumptions, beliefs, and worldviews of nursing education and practice requirements. The most productive conversations on this topic avoid educational-level absolutes. Health improvement concepts require broader discussions beyond a sole emphasis on the degree conferred. Leaders can stimulate movement toward an integration of health science education to achieve a foundation of shared meaning, skills, and language that leads to various practice fields or disciplines but keeps sight of the common link of service rather than reinforcement of discipline-specific needs. This foundation may eventually help to blur the discipline boundaries that do not serve consumer needs.

The model shift also identifies that nursing education curriculum revision is required to address current and anticipated needs for different skills while retaining the traditional interest on care for the whole person in the family and community context. Education revision leads to reassessment of licensure issues to assure that licensure meets public needs and not discipline needs. Planning based on such assessment avoids another self-induced shortage of nurses due to short-term, nonadaptive actions.

The conversation regarding demand for nurses in managed care environments is as complex as the care delivery system itself. The long-term benefit of managed care systems may be the rethinking of the nature of service and service delivery in health care and the eventual development of the type and number of providers needed for this new era.

ACKNOWLEDGMENTS

My appreciation to my colleagues in the expert panel for sharing their expertise and visions for the future: Ruth Kingdon, assistant hospital administrator at Kaiser Foundation Hospital in Fontana, California; Julie Morath, system vice president, quality and clinical care improvement for Allina Health System in Minneapolis; Mary Ross, vice president of Presbyterian Healthcare Services in

Albuquerque; Eileen Sporing, vice president of Children's Hospital in Boston; the members of the Allina Patient Care Council in Minneapolis-St. Paul; and my colleagues at United Hospital in St. Paul.

References

Aroskar, M. "Managed Care and Nursing Values: A Reflection." *Trends in Health Care, Law, & Ethics,* 1995, *10,* Winter-Spring, 83–86.

Finocchio, L. J., Dower, C. M., McMahon, T., Gragnola, C. M., and the Taskforce on Health Care Workforce Regulation. *Reforming Health Care Workforce Regulation: Policy Considerations for the 21st Century.* San Francisco: UCSF Center for the Health Professions, 1995.

Goldsmith, J., Goran, M., and Nackel, J. "Managed Care Comes of Age." *Healthcare Forum Journal,* 1995, Sept.-Oct., 14–24.

Halvorsen, G. *Strong Medicine.* New York: Random House, 1993.

Heifetz, R. *Leadership Without Easy Answers.* Cambridge, Mass.: Belknap Press, 1994.

Hicks, L., Stallmeyer, J., and Coleman, J. "Nursing Challenges in Managed Care." *Nursing Economics,* 1992, July-Aug., 265–276.

Lindeman, C. "Changing Vision to Reality: Preparing Tomorrow's Nurses." Keynote address, Minnesota League for Nursing, Mar. 8, 1995.

Madison, D., and Konrad, T. "Large Medical Group-Practice Organizations and Employed Physicians: A Relationship in Transition." *Milbank Memorial Quarterly,* 1988, *66*(2), 240–282.

Minnesota Organization of Leaders in Nursing, 1664 N.W. 17th Street, St. Paul, Minn. 55112–5466. Position paper, May 1996.

Newman, M. "Toward an Integrative Model of Professional Practice." *Journal of Professional Nursing,* 1990, *6,* May-June, 167–173.

United HealthCare Corporation. *The Language of Managed Care and Organized Health Care Systems.* Minnetonka, Minn.: United Health Care Corporation, 1994.

Article List: Environmental Assessment

Compiled by Maureen Swan, Allina Health System

Abramowitz, K. *The Future of Health Care Delivery in America,* Oct. 27, 1995.

American Association of Health Plans. *Executive Summary: Industry Positioning Campaign,* Feb. 1996.

American Hospital Association. *Health Care Fact File,* Aug. 1995.

American Medical Association. "Practices Sell, Hospitals Lose." *American Medical News,* Dec. 11, 1995.

Avalos, G. "Netscape Founder to Take Health Care On-Line," *Contra Cost Times,* Mar. 8, 1996.

Baumgarten, A. *Minnesota Managed Care Review 1995*, Sept. 1995.

Boston Globe. "Survey Reveals High Quality HMOs May Not Be Most Popular," Apr. 3, 1996.

Bransten, L. "Aetna Purchase Highlights a Growing Trend: Acquisitions of US Healthcare May Create National Managed Care Groups." *The Financial Times*, Apr. 4, 1996.

Brown, M. "Health Care 2015: Flight of the Butterfly." *Physician Executive*, Jan. 1996.

Cerne, F. "Money and Management." *Hospitals and Health Networks*, Jan. 5, 1995.

City Business. *Critical Choices: 1995 Health Care Guide*, 1995.

City of Minneapolis. *Children, Adolescents, and Violence*, 1994.

Commercenet and Nielsen, Inc. *Commercenet/Nielsen Internet Demographics Survey*, 1995.

Dartmouth Medical School, *Dartmouth Atlas of Health Care*, July 5, 1995.

Davis, K., and others. "Choice Matters: Enrollees' Views of Their Health Plans," *Health Affairs*, Summer 1995.

Deloitte & Touche, LLP. *Healthcare Benefits in Minnesota: 1995 Survey Results*, 1995.

Gallup Organization. *The Gallup Organization Public Concerns Poll Newsletter Archive*, 1995.

Gallup Organization. *The Gallup Organization Wish List Newsletter Archive*, 1995.

Goldstein, D. *The Growth of the Physician Practice Management Industry: Background and Financial Issues for Allina Health System*, Apr. 2, 1996.

Health Care Advisory Board. *Emerging from Shadow: Resurgence to Prosperity Under Managed Care*, Washington, D.C., 1995.

Health Care Advisory Board. *Network Advantage*, Washington, D.C., 1995.

Health Care Advisory Board. *The Third Wave of Health Care Cost Savings*, Washington, D.C., 1995.

Health Care Advisory Board. *The Conference Report on Medicaid*, Washington, D.C., Dec. 1995.

Health Care Advisory Board. *Executive Briefing: Resurgence of Choice*, Washington, D.C., 1996.

Heineccius, L. *Columbia/HCA: A National Profile*, Dec. 1, 1995.

Hennepin County Community Health Department. *Summary Report Card on Health Issues*, Fall 1995.

Hennepin County Health Policy Center. *Publicly Funded Health Programs in Hennepin County*, Dec. 1995.

Interstudy. *The Interstudy Competitive Edge: Part II, Industry Report*, Sept. 1995.

Interstudy. *The Interstudy Competitive Edge: Part III, Regional Market Analysis*, Nov. 1995.

Kaiser Family Foundation. *Kaiser Family Foundation Survey on American's Perceptions About For-Profit Health Care*, Dec. 1995.

Kaiser, L. "Health Care In The 21st Century." *Physician Executive,* Jan. 1996.

KPMG Peat Marwick, LLP. *National Managed Care Study,* 1996.

Leutwyler, K. "The Price of Prevention." *Scientific American,* Apr. 1995.

Lewin-VHI, Inc., and NCQA. *Tracking the System: American Health Care 1996,* Feb. 1996.

Little, A. *Challenges of the Managed Care Marketplace,* 1995.

Lutz, S. "Doc Companies Dominate Top IPOs." *Modern Healthcare,* Jan. 22, 1996.

Marion Merrell Dow, Inc. *Managed Care Digest Series: Institutional Digest,* 1995.

McManis, J. *New Marketplace Directions: Shaping Future Healthcare Delivery,* Oct. 1995.

Minnesota Department of Health. *Minnesota Health Care Market Report,* 1995.

Modern Healthcare. "Doc Practice Management Set To Explode," Aug. 14, 1995.

Modern Healthcare. "Kaiser Retools to Fight For Lost Ground," July 17, 1995.

Modern Healthcare. "Outlook 1996," Jan. 1996.

National Research Corporation. *The NRC Healthcare Market Guide: Market Highlights,* 1994.

Newsweek. "Online: Staying Alive," Feb. 12, 1996.

"Outlook 1996." *The Futurist,* World Future Society, 1995.

Physicians Managed Care Report. *Heart Specialists Turn to Networks for Long-Term Stability,* Oct. 1994.

Physicians Services of America. *1995–96 Survey of Physician Salary Expectations,* Oct. 1995.

Post Bulletin. "Electronic Health Guide Updated," Oct. 18, 1995.

Rivo, M., and Kindig, D. "A Report Card on the Physician Work Force in the United States," *New England Journal of Medicine,* Apr. 4, 1996.

Sachs Group, Inc. *Consumers and Their Health Plans: National Summary,* Nov. 1995.

Star Tribune. "Alternative Therapies," Oct. 17, 1995.

Star Tribune. "Minnesota Poll," Feb. 1996.

Star Tribune. "On the Edge of the Digital Age," June 1995.

Star Tribune. "Study: Doctor, Chiropractor Backache Results Equal," Oct. 5, 1995.

Tomsho, R. "Free Agent Doctors Are Selling Practices, Signing Job Contracts." *Wall Street Journal,* Mar. 12, 1996.

Towers, P. *Navigating the Changing Health Care System: The Towers Perrin Survey of What Americans Know and Need to Know,* 1995.

United Way of the Minneapolis Area. *The Face of the Twin Cities: Another Look. Trends Affecting Our Community Through 2000,* 1995.

VHA/Deloitte & Touche, Allina Health System. *Health Gain: Improving the Health of Communities Through Integrated Healthcare,* 1994.

VHA/Deloitte & Touche. *New Roles, New Responsibilities For Health: Responding to Imperatives For Change,* 1996.

Weil, T., and Jorgensen, N. "Health Manpower Trends in a Market-Driven Environment," *Journal of Healthcare Resource Management,* Dec. 1995.

"Who Has Too Many Beds?" *Hospitals and Health Networks,* Jan. 5, 1996.

CHAPTER FIVE

How Is Demand for Registered Nurses in Hospital Settings Changing?

Maryann F. Fralic

The next four chapters focus on changes in RNs' roles and demand for their services in specific health care delivery settings. This segment of the book begins with the hospital, which, despite the increased shift of care delivery to other settings, continues to employ the largest number of RNs. With the arrival of the market in health care, the hospital moves from being a highly valued revenue center to the focus of cost control, forcing it to examine the processes associated with the delivery of care and to adapt to patients who are, on average, more acutely ill. This has led to an increase in demand for advanced practice nurses and expanded use of ancillary personnel in support of nursing service. Further research on nurse staffing models is needed to ascertain which models are most effective. Fralic concludes that the supply of nursing professionals is adequate to meet the requirements of hospitals in the near term, with respect to absolute numbers of RNs. She does, however, point to the need to prepare more nurses at the baccalaureate level to meet the more complicated needs of patients. As the workplace and technology supporting nursing practice change, nurses will increasingly be under pressure to differentiate the practice of associate- and baccalaureate-prepared RNs. This will mean significant changes in the hospital team and the deployment of nurses to outpatient units. Ultimately the role of the hospital and hospital-based nurses will be determined as the institution and the profession can demonstrate their efficacy in delivery of highly valued services, as compared to alternative sources of care. To be successful in such an environment will require the nursing profession to fully understand and to help lead the transition in health care.

Nursing practice in hospitals cannot be separated from its societal, political, economic, and organizational context. Chapter One outlines the broad parameters within which hospitals are changing, but further detail is essential to understanding the specific implications of these changes for hospital-based nursing.

THE NEW CONTEXT OF NURSING PRACTICE IN HOSPITALS

The context of contemporary hospitals is chaotic indeed. As Keegan describes (1994), hospitals are quickly evolving from being highly valued revenue centers to being very expensive cost centers. This singular transformation is quite profound in terms of its impact on shaping the context of health care. With the increased movement to global billing schemes, predetermined fixed payment, and deeply discounted capitation, hospitals are increasingly becoming financial risk-bearing organizations.

Tightly capitated environments cause every patient intervention and action to be closely scrutinized as to cost and effectiveness. Individual elements of patient care no longer generate revenue as in traditional reimbursement systems. For example, in the past each physical therapy treatment, each laboratory test, each day in a critical care unit generated incremental revenue. Now each represents an additional expense. A profound change.

These developments create an inexorable movement by hospitals to re-form the processes of clinical care. The models of yesterday and today are simply not designed to meet stringent externally imposed new standards for cost and quality. With growing accountability for the cost and quality of care across sites, across a continuum of care, and often across a lifetime, the true interdependency of hospitals with other care settings becomes apparent. Hospital care takes on complex added dimensions, at times organizing around specialty practice or defined centers of excellence. There is a new focus on effectiveness and efficiency, quality and cost, and the timely achievement and quantification of specific clinical and financial outcomes. There is an urgency to reduce the unit cost of care, to consistently recreate clinical processes, and to critically evaluate the fundamental organization of patient care. New areas of responsibility put unfamiliar burdens on hospital staff and require new approaches that are both relevant and responsive to the rapid changes in health care.

In this context, only the most acutely ill persons with the most serious illnesses will be admitted to hospitals. While payment for these services decreases, expectations for outcomes grow. Technological advances heighten the complexity of hospital care, which has led to higher levels of acuity within the hospital and strong pressure to continually move patients to less acute settings. The common prediction that hospitals will become large critical care units is not unwarranted. As patients are moved out of critical care beds more quickly, that level of patient acuity is transferred to the general medical-surgical units. As a result, the patients in today's subacute care units and in some nursing homes very much resemble yesterday's general hospital patients. One can foresee hospitals with almost rapid-fire patient throughput, a constant deceleration of the average length of stay, escalating intensity, and even higher degrees of specialization.

As one examines the increasing concentration of high intensity of illness in hospitals, the changes in requirements for nursing care are obvious. As Aiken notes (1995, p. 201), "When the current frenzy to restructure slows down, the presence of increasingly ill patients in hospitals will necessitate even higher nurse-to-patient ratios." And more complex patient populations will require better-prepared nurses. This becomes quite obvious as we look at the fundamental change in the nature of hospital care.

This is the highly dynamic backdrop against which acute care nursing work-force requirements must be examined. What types of nurses, in what mix, in what numbers, and at what levels of education can meet these challenges?

SUPPLY AND DEMAND FOR RNS

Predicting workforce requirements in a stable state environment is relatively safe and straightforward. In those circumstances, one only needs to examine the hospital segment of the health care industry, study existing models and statistics within that industry, add normal trends moving forward, and then define future needs in order to achieve a fairly high level of accuracy. However, when projecting a future that is undefined and rapidly evolving from the basis of a constantly changing present, the task is daunting. To examine how many RNs will be needed for future hospital settings requires an assessment of current patterns of use combined with a model of how hospitals, their utilization, and their employment of RNs will change in the future. The second part of this task is problematic.

This chapter highlights only studies of particular relevance to future demand for RNs in hospital settings. An in-depth review of recent forecasts of demand for RNs is provided in Chapter Three. (See Figure 3.2 for a graphical display of projections.)

Data from the past decade indicate that the decrease in hospital utilization has yet to result in a decline in aggregate RN employment in hospitals. To the contrary, Figure 5.1 shows that the number of full-time equivalent RNs employed by community hospitals increased by approximately 30 percent between 1985 and 1994, despite an approximately 10 percent decrease in the number of hospital beds. As noted in Chapter Two, this trend probably reflects both increased patient acuity and a shift in RN positions from inpatient to outpatient units within hospitals.

Two studies consider the impact of managed care on demand for RNs in hospitals. Buerhaus and Staiger (1996) report strong overall growth in RN employment (37 percent) from 1983 to 1994. However, they also found that states with

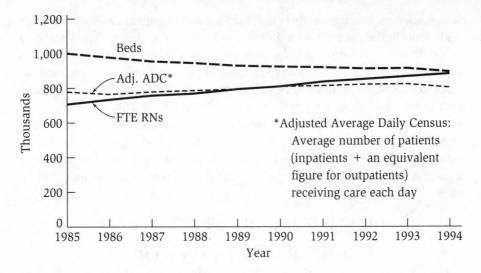

Figure 5.1. Full-Time Equivalent Registered Nurses Employed in Community Hospitals, 1985–1994.

Source: American Hospital Association, 1995

high HMO enrollment experience slower RN employment growth in hospitals. This likely reflects lower hospital utilization rates in high HMO enrollment states. These findings suggest that overall growth in RN employment will slow as overall HMO enrollment increases.

A phenomenon to follow in hospitals will be the change in utilization of nurses per bed, as patient intensity continues to escalate. A Public Policy Institute of California study (Spetz, 1996) specifically examined the change in number of hours worked by hospital nursing personnel. California data are important because it is a bellwether state with one of the highest rates of HMO enrollment in the nation. The study reported "a steady increase in the number of hours worked by nursing personnel over the past eighteen years. Most of the growth resulted from an increase in the number of hours worked by registered nurses; the use of licensed vocational nurses and nursing aides has declined or remained stable. In addition to total hours, the hours worked by nursing personnel per hospital discharge and per patient day have risen, indicating that more nursing resources are serving patients admitted to hospitals in California" (p. iii). This study further reported that in 1977 RNs worked about four hours per patient day, but in 1995 more than eight hours per patient day (p. 9).

Based on these and other studies of trends in supply and demand for RNs, this chapter stakes out the middle ground, projecting that the overall supply of registered nurses will be generally adequate into the next century in terms of absolute numbers of RNs. This projection incorporates the downsizing of the hospital sector, but also predicts that the increase in patient case mix intensity and comorbidity coupled with a decrease in length of stay within acute care hospitals will increase demand for RNs to a level that will fully offset the effects of downsizing. It is acknowledged that the educational mix of nurses remains a pernicious problem and will be carried forward, absent any corrective strategies to increase the number of RNs educated at the baccalaureate level. These conclusions are consistent with those reached by the members of the Institute of Medicine committee on nurse staffing in hospitals and nursing homes (Institute of Medicine, 1996), whose recommendations are displayed in Table 5.1, as well as those of other nursing workforce experts (Aiken and Salmon, 1994).

THE NEW WORK, THE NEW TECHNOLOGY, AND THE IMPACT ON DEMAND

The genesis and focus of reengineering efforts in hospitals over the last five to ten years reflect the context of patient care in hospitals during this period. There were generally many registered nurses, very few assistive personnel, a stable patient population, and a relatively leisurely (by today's standards) length of stay. All of this made it perfectly natural to reengineer with an emphasis on eliminating large numbers of registered nurses and replacing them with large numbers of lower-skilled assistive personnel. This fit the patient population at that time and seemed to be an appropriate direction. Today, however, with a compressed patient stay, incredible increases in technology, and a very high level of patient acuity, the old reengineering model no longer works.

Emerging patterns of hospital care require highly trained and highly skilled registered nurses. Consider, for example, what goes on during a one-day stay for a radical mastectomy patient (many would have considered this unthinkable not long ago). The sheer volume and criticality of the interventions for that patient during that day make the case. It is not a situation where a nurse can occasionally see the patient, directing other levels of staff to care for her. Rather, you have a clinically intense hospital stay, with the overlay of emotion and high anxiety that typically accompanies this surgery, and yet the patient is scheduled to go home that night. You therefore need a nurse with very keen assessment skills, the ability to conduct almost moment-by-moment analysis of the patient's progress, with analytic assessment followed by prompt and appropriate clinical intervention. In addition to caring for the patient, the nurse is also managing a copious amount of technical equipment such as tubes, drains, parenteral fluids, pain control equipment, and often physiologic monitoring devices. This patient also requires comprehensive pre- and posthospital planning and intervention. All of this must be very well coordinated.

Table 5.1. Recommendations on Staffing and Quality in Hospitals.

Recommendation: The committee recommends that hospitals expand the use of RNs with advance practice preparation and skills to provide clinical leadership and cost-effective patient care, particularly for patients with complex management problems.

Recommendation: The committee recommends that hospitals have documented evidence that ancillary nursing personnel are competent and that such personnel are tested and certified by an appropriate entity for this competence. The committee further recommends that the training for ancillary nursing personnel working in hospitals be structured and enriched by including training of the following types: appropriate clinical care of the aged and disabled; occupational health and safety measures; culturally sensitive care; and appropriate management of conflict.

Recommendation: The committee recommends that hospital leaders involve nursing personnel (RNs, Licensed Practical Nurses, and Nurse Assistants) who are directly affected by organizational redesign and staffing reconfiguration in the process of planning and implementing such changes.

Recommendation: The committee recommends that hospital management monitor and evaluate the effects of changes in organizational redesign and reconfiguration of nursing personnel on patient outcomes, on patient satisfaction, and on nursing personnel themselves.

Recommendation: The committee recommends that the National Institute of Nursing Research (NINR) and other appropriate agencies fund scientifically sound research on the relationships between quality of care and nurse staffing levels and mix, taking into account organization variables. The committee further recommends that NINR, along with the Agency for Health Care Policy and Research (AHCPR) and private organizations, develop a research agenda on quality of care.

Recommendation: The committee recommends that an interdisciplinary public-private partnership be organized to develop performance and outcome measures that are sensitive to nursing interventions and care, with uniform definitions that are measurable in a uniform manner across all hospitals.

Source: Reprinted with permission from *Nurse Staffing in Hospitals and Homes: Is it Adequate?,* National Academy Press, 1996.

Some areas of the country are designing an eight-day hospital length of stay for heart transplant patients and three-day length of stay for renal transplant patients. Length of stay is also declining for many other conditions. Reduced length of stay per patient requires increased activity per patient per day. The concentration and nature of that activity drives nursing work. For example, when a patient was hospitalized for a total of eight days for open heart surgery, the pace of care, interventions, and activity for that patient was reasonably staged and planned each day. Today, in markets with high managed care enrollment rates, that length of stay is three or four days for the same procedure, and the pace of activity per patient per day more than doubles. And just as hospitals plan to respond to these requirements, endoscopic closed heart surgery is now being performed, further reducing the hospital stay to two days.

These scenarios will increasingly become more commonplace. Therefore, hospitals will require seasoned registered nurses with high levels of skill and competency to manage these patient populations. It is not simply a matter of "doing the tasks." This registered nurse should be well prepared both educationally and experientially if the patient is to have a successful outcome and meet established clinical outcomes and length-of-stay targets.

As ever more complicated technology is introduced into clinical settings, nurses must acquire and master the skills to manage that technology. Paradoxically, advances in technology can both compound and alleviate the challenges of providing nursing care in hospitals. New technology and sophisticated equipment often require additional nursing time. The sheer amount, intricacy, and criticality of equipment at the patient's bedside add to the nursing workload. An excellent illustration is the highly technical bedside machine for continuous venous to venous hemofiltration (CVVH) for critically ill patients with multi-system disease. This technology is an extremely effective clinical treatment modality. However, it increases the demand for highly skilled nurses, often requiring a constant 1:1 nurse-patient ratio. This is one of many clear illustrations that even as hospital beds decrease in overall numbers, the nurse requirements per bed will tend to increase in response to a concentrated high-acuity patient population. This will modify the otherwise natural decline in nurse requirements that typically accompanies hospital downsizing.

Yet much of this technology will indeed save nursing time. For example, new optical scanner technology allows for online arterial blood gas monitoring; new central monitoring hubs can track multiple physiological parameters. Chapter One rightly highlights the critical role of information systems. Thoughtfully designed, automated documentation systems can eliminate tedious paper-and-pencil charting that nurses have historically done. Computerized "nurse finder" features on newly released patient call systems can locate nurses promptly and silently, dispatching them quickly to locations where they are needed.

Clearly the steady incorporation of new technology into patient care settings needs to be closely evaluated for both positive and negative impact on nurse staffing. In turn, nursing administrators and educators must ensure that RNs have the competencies needed to use new technologies effectively.

It is clear from all empirical, anecdotal, and factual data that the overall number of acute care hospitals will decrease in the future, and those that remain will continue to become smaller in size, with fewer beds but with a greater concentration of patient acuity per bed. As hospital admission requirements become ever more stringent, the intensity of care requirements per patient will continue to grow.

So the pace continues to quicken and targets are constantly redefined. Every clinical target and critical element of care must be met, every patient outcome must be achieved, and all within a very truncated hospital stay. With each fraction of a day of length-of-stay reduction, patient activities further concentrate. The combination of decreasing hospital days, more acutely ill patients, and the ever-increasing sophistication and concentration of the elements of patient care is inexorably altering the requirements for RNs.

NEW MODELS FOR PATIENT CARE/DIFFERENTIATING PRACTICE

Every health care organization is under extreme pressure to deliver affordable and high-quality patient care, yet it is increasingly difficult to meet these requirements with existing patient care models. Simply retrofitting yesterday's models will not and cannot be right for tomorrow's challenges. Fresh approaches to clinical care must be created to minimize cost, increase efficiency, and enhance quality. These models must focus on the patient. Registered nurses have the opportunity—and the responsibility—to help design the high-quality care delivery systems for tomorrow's patients.

Approaches to staffing in this new environment will be extremely diverse, with many new designs implemented within individual hospitals and across hospital systems. As the number of multihospital integrated delivery systems increases, more and more nurses are being cross-trained to work in several hospitals to address fluctuations in the staffing needs of individual hospitals. Some new models are designed so that nurses are hired within an entire system and are able to work in various member hospitals. For example, this is true of the largest for-profit hospital chain, which hires a cadre of nurses to staff various hospitals nationally where needed. Cross-training between acute care and home care within a single system is a variation of that approach that adds to nurses' skill base and creates more professional flexibility in the process. Staffing patterns such as these will increase demand for nurses who are broadly competent, highly skilled, and professionally confident and comfortable moving within systems and across systems, always responding to the changing requirements of patient populations.

Nurses also will need to function effectively within the nursing team in hospitals. The nursing team is composed of nurses prepared at various levels: licensed practical and vocational, associate degree, baccalaureate degree, and advanced practice nurses. Each level brings its own set of specific skills to the practice setting, and the utilization of each level will depend on the choice of each organization and the context of the practice setting. The majority of hospitals also successfully employ assistive personnel (nonlicensed staff who provide valuable supportive services) as members of nursing teams to expand and leverage the time of RNs. They are best utilized to replace the time that nurses have traditionally spent on tasks that unlicensed personnel could perform, given adequate training and supervision.

This emphasis on cross-training and team delivery of care has focused new attention on the concept of differentiating practice within groups of nurses according to educational levels. Effective teamwork requires that all members are assigned responsibilities commensurate with their education and experience. As Koerner (1992) observes, "If nursing is to meet the demands of a rapidly changing health care system, care delivery models that differentiate scope of job responsibility based on education, experience, and competence must be developed. This will be a transitional, yet crucial step in the development of professional nursing that will maximize cost and quality outcomes for clients and healthcare organizations" (p. 37).

Stilwell's observations (1995, p. 6) about nursing practice in many countries further demonstrate the need for differentiation:

> The uniqueness of nursing practice lies in the ability of the nurse to integrate all of the domains of nursing practice in a way which is responsive to the needs of individuals, families and groups, which will therefore be different for each situation. The truly expert nurse will be able to use a wide range of competencies within each domain, while the naivest practitioner, or the health care assistant with only a limited knowledge base, will not possess all the competencies in each domain and will function in a less flexible way. Expert nursing practice is built on knowledge, experience and the ability to reflect on, and research, practice.

Stilwell is distinguishing between types and levels of nurses and highlights the expert, who is practicing from a broad and deep knowledge base in nursing and who demonstrates creativity and innovation, deals with uncertainty, and is able to research, develop, and expand nursing practice. She states that "these differences in levels of practice may be echoed in educational qualifications" (p. 6).

Many additional observers, professionals, and health care organizations have recommended differentiating nursing practice by level of education (Aiken and

Salmon, 1994; Koerner, 1992; Institute of Medicine, 1996; Moses, 1994; Pew Health Professions Commission, 1995). Hospitals are utilizing nurses with a more expansive educational base to care for their highly complex patient populations. Baccalaureate nurses bring value in the clinical management of more acutely ill and complex patient populations. As the need for analytic and evaluative skill increases at the bedside, baccalaureate nurses will be utilized more frequently. Present market conditions account for hospitals selecting baccalaureate nurses for staff nurse roles in hospitals in increasing numbers over lesser-prepared nurses. With little or no difference in salaries, employers are selecting the best-prepared nurses when given the opportunity.

Meanwhile, some hospitals, such as the Johns Hopkins Hospital, are now utilizing associate degree nurses in more circumscribed technical roles in new care delivery models. At Hopkins, they function with differentiated accountabilities and responsibilities, as delineated in position descriptions. For example, bachelors of science in nursing (BSNs) and associate degree nurses (ADNs) will differ in their practice in the areas of span and scope of practice, degree of autonomy, care coordination responsibilities, management of others' performance, delegatory scope, nursing research and application, and participation in the analysis and utilization of clinical and financial data. Baccalaureate and associate degree nurses each have valuable contributions to make to patient care and can be incorporated very effectively into care models, reflecting their skill level and educational preparation.

Differentiating nursing practice according to levels of education is very timely for new health care environments. Aiken and Salmon (1994) have concluded that the United States is producing too few BSNs and APNs and too many ADNs. As noted in Chapter Two, Division of Nursing statistics show that in 1996 almost 60 percent of all RNs were prepared at less than the baccalaureate level. The division's projections state that by the year 2020, 51.4 percent of all nurses will still continue to be prepared at less than the baccalaureate level, absent any intervention (National Advisory Council on Nursing Education and Practice, 1996). At present there are no substantive differentiating outcomes and performance expectations for nursing graduates of the various schools, and very few exist in the practice setting. It is as though we assume that a 100 percent difference in length of education makes no difference. This must change if we are to meet the requirements of patients in tomorrow's hospital settings.

The nursing workforce as it is constituted today cannot meet tomorrow's requirements. Nurses that deliver patient care in tomorrow's hospitals will increasingly require delegation skills, group management skills, clinical management skills, resilience, high energy, high technical task capability, and analytic and cognitive capability. Critical thinking and higher levels of professional judgment and autonomy will be essential, requiring that a preponderance of baccalaureate-educated nurses be prepared.

The American Association of Colleges of Nursing has established detailed standards (1986) for baccalaureate education in nursing. To properly coordinate care, the professional nurse must demonstrate "the ability to conceptualize the total continuing health care needs for the patient/client and the impact of critical issues including legal and ethical aspects of care" (p. 14). "The nurse applies knowledge and research findings to practice and raises questions for further research about how practice should be conducted in changing health care environments" (p. 16).

Primm (1987) describes the nurse with a BSN as caring for patients who have multiple nursing diagnoses and require complex interactions. Their area of practice includes both structured and unstructured health care settings. The BSN manages comprehensive nursing care, identifying needs from admission to post-discharge (p. 222). The ADN is described as caring for patients who have common well-defined nursing diagnoses, functioning in a structured health care setting that is a geographical or situational environment with established policies, procedures, and protocols (p. 222).

Baccalaureate-prepared nurses will provide leadership for direct patient care, utilizing teams of multiskilled staff. A future-oriented model of care must accommodate the rapid throughput of patients while achieving desired clinical outcomes. Teams must be created that are affordable, acknowledging that patient care in hospital organizations must be both high quality and cost-competitive. Therefore, due diligence must be paid to the development of new care models, considering adequacy of educational levels of staff, differentiation of practice, attention to competency and skill mix, and appropriate levels of compensation. And the composition of the team must—first and foremost—match the clinical requirements of the patient population.

Another important element of differentiated practice will be the development of appropriate roles for advanced practice nurses (APNs) in hospitals. Advanced practice nurse utilization is growing rapidly because these nurses bring master's level preparation, competence, and a solid experience base to clinical settings. Figure 5.2 illustrates this growth. APNs are particularly adept at managing patients with complicated clinical situations and can skillfully plan for care across time and place. These strengths will be highly valued in the new hospital environments. Advanced practice nurses who function as nurse practitioners and case managers are being utilized in rapidly growing numbers in hospitals, creating new demands for these nurses. In some hospitals they function independently while in others they lead nursing teams.

Together these various types of nursing personnel will compose contemporary nursing teams. Their talents can blend and complement each other to provide clinical care that is high quality at an affordable cost. The type and number of staff will be situational and will vary by organization. Multiskilled and cross-trained staff will be essential at all levels, from professionals to assistive per-

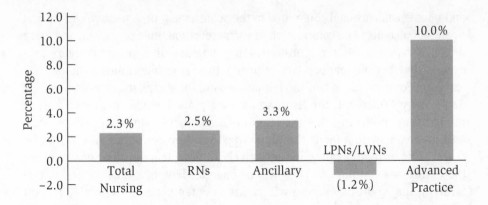

Figure 5.2. U.S. Nursing Personnel: Percentage Change by Category, September 1994–1995.

Source: American Hospital Association, 1995

sonnel. Work should be differentiated and compensation determined according to levels of preparation and accountability. These will be hallmark characteristics of the effective hospital nursing staff of tomorrow.

CHARACTERISTICS OF THE NEW MULTIDISCIPLINARY CARE TEAM IN HOSPITALS

In addition to working effectively within nursing teams, nurses in hospitals will need to be productive members of larger multidisciplinary teams that plan and manage patient care. One can no longer examine each profession in isolation, trying to calculate the impact of each individual profession on patient outcomes. Patient care is simply too fast-paced, complex, and multivariate.

The Joint Commission on Accreditation of Healthcare Organizations (1996) emphasizes the concept of the health care team. It surveys hospitals for evidence that various disciplines plan, deliver, and evaluate patient care together. Acutely ill patient populations, with truncated high-intensity hospital stays, require that the health care team of the future work together in very different ways indeed. The predominant theme will be the concept of highly effective collaboration between professions and new relationships among the various health care disciplines. Old methods simply will not work. All team members together must identify and plan approaches that maximize efficient resource utilization and facilitate optimal patient outcomes.

The effective care team of the future will be multiprofessional, highly interactive, and collaborative, recognizing and valuing each discipline's contribution and interdependence and committed to the achievement of aggressive clinical and financial outcomes. The contribution of each profession must be valued, and every person's expertise drawn upon to develop patient-oriented care delivery processes. Together the team creates critical pathways or algorithms to guide clinical care. For example, when the reimbursement for a cardiac surgery procedure declines by 10 percent, the team adjusts the plan. Then, a further change in reimbursement dictates that the length of stay must go down by another day, and the team again adjusts the plan. Together they determine how it can be done. They respond swiftly and effectively to new demands and can improve their processes continually. They will be energized by the challenge and uncertainty in the environment and will create new templates for effective patient care management.

Advanced practice nurses will increasingly become key members of these teams, causing demand for them to rise even further. An important element of their new work is becoming an effective member of the team, leading in some situations and following in others. These nurses will be skilled as interdisciplinary collaborators, standard setters, and outcomes monitors, able to plan across continuums of care and design new approaches to management of clinical care.

Many questions emerge when one contemplates how physicians, nurses, and other professionals will build and sustain effective teams. What is the right mix of health care providers for these new patient care systems and new patient populations? How will each discipline be prepared and how will they interrelate? How can the professions be socialized to work together, sharing classes and course work as team members throughout their educational process? This raises questions as to whether it is appropriate or desirable to perpetuate insular and parallel processes for the preparation and practice of key interdependent health care professions. As we reengineer core processes in hospitals and in health care, should we also be reengineering the composition, the educational processes, the function, and the evaluative processes of the new health care team?

MEASUREMENT, EVALUATION, AND RESEARCH OPPORTUNITIES

The new work of registered nurses in hospitals will also include the requirement to share accountability with other disciplines for clinical and financial outcomes. This may take the form of coordinating care according to critical pathways, participating in the definition and achievement of specific patient outcomes, and planning for both pre- and posthospital care. And there is the need to match clinical practice and interventions day by day with preprogrammed plans of care and then to document and respond to variances in practice. All of these activities are new and they require thorough evaluation and research.

As contemporary models of care are planned, keen attention must be given to creating evaluation research plans so that evaluation is integral to the design and not an afterthought. Without data, effectiveness cannot be determined.

Concurrent measurement provides for utilization of new care models as learning laboratories, offering the opportunity for ongoing refinement and adaptation. Evaluation research provides the database and effectiveness tracking by which to match the appropriate numbers and levels of registered nurses and other care delivery personnel to the needs of patient populations. Today's dramatic changes in hospitals present extraordinary research opportunities to examine the clinical and financial effectiveness of various nurse staffing models.

Many informed observers note the dearth of research on the relationship between staffing mix and patient outcomes. The Institute of Medicine's study (1996) reports that "there is a serious paucity of recent research on the definitive effects of structural measures, such as specific staffing ratios, on the quality of patient care in terms of patient outcomes when controlling for all other likely explanatory or confounding variables. . . . Across-the-board staffing ratios tend to assume that in some measure all patients are 'alike' and can be cared for with the same level and type of resources. Equally difficult is the task of establishing ratios that will be appropriate for all settings and situations" (p. 121).

Determining staffing levels has been rather perfunctory in the past. But yesterday's methods of determining staffing requirements cannot apply in today's fast-paced, high-intensity hospitals. Formerly, the midnight census and a general acuity system constituted an adequate information and decision support base. Today, a more comprehensive approach to staffing configuration is required.

To design and staff new care models, more data-intensive and rigorous methods are required. Table 5.2 depicts the elements considered in developing staffing plans for the Patient Care Delivery Model for The Johns Hopkins Hospital. These elements permit customization of staffing formats for each individual patient care unit, reflecting the needs of specific patient populations.

It is evident that far more than midnight census and generic patient acuity systems are needed for proper calculation of staffing needs. One element, for example, proves crucial. The admission-discharge-transfer (ADT) index is pivotal to determining the numbers and types of nurses and other care team members required. In the past, one would develop a staffing plan for a thirty-bed unit. Yet in today's hectic hospital environments, a telemetry unit may have a 50 percent ADT index; that is, fifteen more patients per day are processed in that thirty-bed base. So in actuality the care team must be configured so that forty-five patients can be properly cared for within twenty-four hours. That is indeed a dramatic change from yesterday's world, when patients (and staff) enjoyed what now seems to be a leisurely length of stay. Therefore staffing methodologies and nurse workforce allocation must also change. Faculty and students in graduate programs in nursing administration will need to learn contemporary staffing methods.

Table 5.2. A Contemporary Approach to Staffing Configurations.

Nurse staffing decisions were historically based on the traditional measures of midnight census and patient acuity. Expanded analysis assures objective, rigorous, and data-based staffing calculations.

- Work Activity/Analysis Per Unit
  ⇒ Admissions/Discharge/Transfer (ADT) Activity Index
  ⇒ Average Daily Census (ADC)
  ⇒ Time pattern of events/activity
  ⇒ Unit Geography

- Patient Acuity/Case Mix Intensity
  ⇒ Retrospective and concurrent data review
  ⇒ Programmatic changes (planned or projected)
  ⇒ Unit observations/work analysis
  ⇒ Nurse Manager/staff interviews
  ⇒ Level of homogeneity/differentiation of patient populations and physician staff

- Task Complexity Index
  ⇒ Level of Technology (present, planned, projected)
  ⇒ Unit observations/work analysis
  ⇒ Nurse manager/staff interviews

- Level of Support Services
  ⇒ Adequacy/Ability to respond to patient/unit requirements
  ⇒ Nurse Manager/staff interviews
  ⇒ Comparative staffing ratios across clinical services

- Work Force/Staff Mix/Competency
  ⇒ Benchmark and other comparative data
  ⇒ Staffing requirements
  ⇒ Staff level/mix comparisons across clinical services
  ⇒ Licensure/regulatory requirements
  ⇒ Labor force analysis/availability/cost
  ⇒ Staff experience level/competency level

- **Financial Feasibility Studies (serial modeling per unit and per service)**

Reprinted with permission. All rights reserved by Dr. Maryann F. Fralic, the Johns Hopkins Hospital, 1996.

Nurses currently serving as managers and administrators will need to acquire and incorporate new methods for accurate allocation of staff.

Lawrenz & Associates, Inc., prepared a study (1994) that examined length of stay reduction and impact on the hours of care per patient day. This was a self-described nonscientific study of nine hospitals in various geographic regions, and certain findings were of particular interest. One observation was that for each day that length of stay is decreased, approximately one hour per patient per day was increased on general medical-surgical units. Another finding was that increased activity per twenty-four hours—in terms of numbers of admissions, discharges, and transfers—will increase nursing workload profoundly, even if patient care requirements do not change. This results in the need for more nursing time per bed per twenty-four hours, thereby increasing nursing workforce requirements. The Lawrenz report also proposes that higher hours of care may be cost-effective if the overall cost of care per admission (unit cost) is reduced. The importance of the calculation of unit cost has been raised by others and deserves careful study.

As stated previously, when such dramatic levels of change are occurring, an evaluation plan is crucial. The plan must assess the overall effectiveness of a care delivery model, taking into account staff numbers and composition. Clinical outcomes, cost incomes, the impact on efficiency and productivity, the ability to meet service standards, the unit cost per admission, and patient and staff satisfaction are essential elements to be tracked and measured. As with any new intervention, careful preimplementation baseline data must be collected, as well as postimplementation measurement at specific intervals.

These are examples of some of the new challenges facing hospital nursing leadership as staffing plans are calculated and as requirements for the numbers and types of nurses are delineated. The next logical step will be to incorporate hospital data with integrated systems data to study populations of patients across settings, examining entire episodes of illness. It is then possible to arrive at a more comprehensive depiction of patient outcomes on a pre- , post- , and intrahospital basis. Nurses will have increasingly important roles in this longitudinal examination of the effectiveness of clinical care.

IMPLICATIONS FOR NURSING EDUCATION, TRAINING, AND RETRAINING

Three major trends affect the preparation of the nursing workforce for practice in the hospital of the twenty-first century: the rising age of the current workforce and of new graduates, curricular content offered in traditional educational preparation of RNs, and retraining for a restructured health care delivery system.

Chapters Two and Three describe the steady increase in the average age of RNs, an increase driven by both general demographic trends and a rise in the average age at which RNs enter practice. (In particular, see Figure 2.4.) The seemingly inexorable rise in the average age of the nurse is indeed a cause for concern (Institute of Medicine, 1996; National League for Nursing, 1995). Nursing practice is very demanding, hard work physically, intellectually, and emotionally. The intensified pace, workload, and rotating shift assignments in the hospital sector compound these demands.

Any experienced nurse executive knows that the demographics of nurses in hospitals show that the majority of staff nurses are in their twenties and thirties, with a rather predictable drop-off at or around age forty. The latest available data show that the average age of RNs in hospitals is 40.8 years (Moses, 1997, p. 21). How will this match with the data for age at entry into practice? Because most nurses are likely to continue coming to hospitals for their first clinical experience, they will encounter highly demanding environments. Other environments, such as home care, can be considered independent practice settings for nurses and are not typically first practice sites for new graduates.

Another important trend is the welcome and steady growth in the numbers of second-career nursing students who already possess baccalaureate or higher degrees in other fields. They come into nursing later in life, often with successful experience and careers in other occupations or professions and an abiding desire to provide meaningful human service. Many bring high energy and enthusiasm and valuable work and life experience. They represent strong potential for new leadership in nursing because they are not typical twenty-year-olds in their first job experience. They bring new capacities for leadership at a time when this is sorely needed in nursing. However, they also come to their first practice setting later in life, many in their thirties, forties, or even fifties. Their maturity, confidence, and dedication are of significant value to the profession, but they will not have the same number of years for available active participation in the nursing workforce.

The dilemma is real. Younger graduates bring the promise of a longer active participation rate in nursing. Older graduates bring more life experience and maturity. We will continue to have both cohort groups graduating from schools of nursing into the future. Nursing will need to wisely merge both groups within the workplace and maximize the strengths of each.

So the trends become clear. Hospitals will continue to attract the bulk of new nursing graduates who will be older and therefore will have shorter overall working lifetimes in the hospital setting. There will be very serious challenges in matching the future nursing workforce with the work demands of the future hospital—and the backdrop for this is the steadily aging general population. So we may experience the confounding demographics of the aging nursing workforce required to care for an aging general population.

The new work of the nurse in hospitals, as described herein, has enormous implications for nursing education. The nursing workforce must have the knowledge and skills necessary to meet the demands of future hospital-based nursing practice. As Aiken observes (1995), even though large numbers of nurses continue to be produced there are serious inadequacies in their type and level of preparation. The number of graduates from basic baccalaureate programs must increase dramatically if nurses are to practice effectively and exert leadership in contemporary institutional care delivery.

Baccalaureate education prepares professional nurses through specific curricular offerings, delineated by the American Association of Colleges of Nursing in its publication *Essentials of College and University Education for Professional Nursing* (1986). This document states that "the professional nurse provides nursing care to individuals, families, groups, and communities along a continuum of health, illness and disability in multiple settings" (p. 9). Thus, students are taught to determine heath status and health needs based on the interpretation of health-related data, utilizing theories and models that guide nursing practice, data collection tools, and techniques of assessment (p. 9).

Key baccalaureate curricular elements also include the ability to evaluate response to therapeutic interventions, methods for measuring goal attainment, and methods for evaluating the quality of nursing practice. The knowledge needed for an analytic approach to patient care is the nursing process, a conceptual model of nursing practice as a means of planning care and solving clinical problems, and sources of information that include clinical data and research findings. To attain the clinical judgment and related skills needed to use data and research findings as a basis for practice, a baccalaureate student must be able to analyze published and unpublished clinical studies, identify areas or problems for study, and participate in evaluation of nursing practice activities (p. 13).

The National Commission on Nursing Implementation Project listed the ability to think logically, analyze critically, and communicate effectively as a requisite knowledge base of the baccalaureate nurse (1990). The commission's report stated that "the professional nurse's scientific background will provide a distinction between observation and inference in scientific investigation" (p. 131). The report also states that "professional nurses will integrate knowledge from liberal education and nursing and apply this knowledge in client situations" (p. 131). Baccalaureate education encompasses complex and unusual or poorly defined health and illness problems and includes the combination of liberal arts, research and scientific content, social and organizational content, community health content, professional content, and leadership content. The didactic and experiential nature of this educational process enables the nurse to work effectively in both structured environments and in those with much more uncertainty. In contrast, "technical nurses are care givers and participants in developing the plan of care for patients with well-defined health or illness problems" (p. 133).

The curriculum from technical nursing education programs is intended to prepare the associate degree nurse to focus on problem solving with usual, well-defined health and illness problems, working in structured environments.

Intraprofessional debate in nursing continues around the baccalaureate versus associate degree issue. Some believe that baccalaureate and associate degree RNs should be treated similarly in the workplace with no differentiation; others argue that differentiation must occur. Still others propose the associate degree for entry into practice, with the professional degree obtained at the master's level. It is clear that many decades after entry-into-practice issues were first raised, consensus continues to elude us.

Buerhaus and Staiger (1996) note that because baccalaureate nursing education programs prepare nurses for acute care, community, and primary care settings, prudent public policy should focus on shifting the capacity of nurse education toward baccalaureate programs. Hess (1996) reports that "meta-analysis of research on differences in the performance of baccalaureate, associate degree, and diploma nurses has identified that baccalaureate nurses are better prepared for a broader range of nursing competencies and perform better in the professional role" (p. 290). However, Hess also wisely observes, "We are entering the 21st Century without consensus on the appropriate system for conveying nursing knowledge" (p. 292). Very true.

Clear differentiation in focus, content, and objectives should characterize the baccalaureate and associate degree educational programs in nursing. Attention should be directed to the proper alignment of the numbers of new nursing graduates that will be needed from the respective educational programs. Interdisciplinary curriculum and joint learning experiences with physicians in training should characterize baccalaureate and higher education. New learning methods and technologies should be employed to enable the incorporation of these additional requirements into an already overcrowded curriculum. Contemporary topics and skills need to be added to nursing curriculum. Didactic and experiential content to educate nurses about new health care systems and managed care tenets is required. The inclusion of experience in managed care environments during the educational process will help to prepare students for these new realities. Existing curriculum should be scrutinized carefully to see if it meets tomorrow's needs, deleting topics or methods that have outlived their usefulness. (Easy to say, hard to do, but essential if education is to truly prepare practitioners for a new era.)

A close working collaboration between the academic and service settings will be absolutely essential if education is to be relevant and responsive to future health care realities. Faculty need to have exposure, experience, and competency in today's fast-paced and demanding clinical environments, so that there is a realistic experiential base to monitor students and guide ongoing curriculum development.

Given our present and projected realities, the educational system must be focused on preparing larger numbers of baccalaureate nurses who can meet the new demands of present and future patient populations. And associate degree nurses should be utilized appropriately in the workplace, maximizing their strengths and contributions. However, one simply cannot equate the two types of preparation. The baccalaureate- and associate-prepared RNs each bring their own value to the delivery of health care. Collectively they represent an essential national health care resource. The task of nursing leadership is to assure that these resources are utilized wisely.

What policy-level decisions are needed to assure that the majority of new nursing graduates are prepared at the baccalaureate level? What initiatives and funding mechanisms will be necessary?

In addition to the basic formal education of nurses, much training occurs within the hospital setting. Preparation for practice in highly technical areas frequently requires protracted orientation. As nurses are assigned to cover additional clinical areas, or to work in member organizations within integrated delivery systems, significant cross-training must occur. This training is typically provided by the employing organization. The need for this training will increase as registered nurses must continually acquire new skill and new competency within work settings. In addition, the constant integration of complex new technology requires training and ongoing testing for competency.

A more difficult question involves the retraining of nurses displaced by institutional downsizing, bed closures, or hospital closing. When such dislocation occurs, who is responsible for retraining nurses for work in other settings? There are obviously no easy answers to these difficult situations. Do nurses bear responsibility for their own professional development and the acquisition of new skills? Or is that the responsibility of the organization that displaced them? Or should the federal government be responsible for retraining displaced nurses? Should federal responsibility, if any, expand to combine the retraining of displaced physicians along with displaced nurses as key health care professionals? Is this appropriate? Inappropriate? Does this impact on the health care needs of the nation? How? What are the policy implications?

CONCLUSION

There are no simple answers to the question of how the demand for RNs in hospital settings will be affected by the rapid, radical, ongoing changes in health care. As Peter Drucker has instructed, it is not necessary to be clairvoyant to know the future; it is only necessary to clearly interpret what has already happened and then project forward the likely consequences of those happenings. That is what this chapter has attempted to do.

Although studies of future supply and demand for RNs differ in their predictions about the overall adequacy of the numbers of RNs, they strongly agree that the educational mix of nurses is not now adequate nor will it be adequate in the future, absent any intervention.

In the new context of nursing practice in hospitals, RNs will work in newly configured nursing teams to deliver care, and in new multidisciplinary teams that are constituted to plan and manage clinical care. The rapid assimilation of significant numbers of advanced practice nurses—in roles such as case managers and nurse practitioners—is recognized as an important parallel trend.

As hospital utilization decreases, there may be the need for additional nursing hours per patient per day, given the concentrated patient acuity, increased clinical intensity, and decreased length of stay that will continue to occur into the foreseeable future.

Hospitals will decrease in size and number in the future, but they will become centers of concentrated complex patient care, many organized around specialty practice or centers of excellence, utilizing large numbers of highly skilled nurses. RNs will play a key role in developing proper configurations for nurse staffing in hospitals and for measurement of clinical processes and outcomes. The myriad changes described in this chapter will dramatically change hospital nursing practice and staffing, and create an impetus for updating nursing education, training, and requirements for retraining. Policy implications for each area must now be examined.

Differentiation between baccalaureate and associate degree education and practice for nurses is both timely and essential. Additionally the aging of the nursing workforce has serious implications not only for hospitals and health care but for society at large.

Despite the many challenges ahead, nursing brings incredible strength, talent, and optimism to address these challenges. The potential for significant contribution by nursing in shaping the future health care system is impressive indeed.

Thoughtful, timely, and targeted strategic initiatives will assure that both the numbers of professional nurses and the educational mix of those nurses will be appropriate for the future. Properly focused and well-developed policy recommendations at the federal level are necessary and must now be carefully formulated and promulgated. This will be essential if nursing is to successfully address the many challenges of the twenty-first century.

References

Aiken, L. H. "Transformation of the Nursing Workforce." *Nursing Outlook,* 1995, *43,* 201–209.

Aiken, L. H., and Salmon, M. E. "Health Care Workforce Priorities: What Nursing Should Do Now." *Inquiry,* 1994, *31,* 318–329.

American Association of Colleges of Nursing. *Essentials of College and University Education for Professional Nursing.* Final Report. Washington, D.C.: American Association of Colleges of Nursing, 1986.

American Hospital Association. *AHA Hospital Statistics: The AHA Profile of United States Hospitals 9/95, 1994–95 Edition. Data Compiled from the American Hospital Association 1993 Annual Survey of Hospitals.* Chicago: American Hospital Association, 1994.

American Hospital Association. Special tabulations from AHA annual surveys, 1983–1993, prepared for the Institute of Medicine Committee on the Adequacy of Nurse Staffing in Hospitals and Nursing Homes. Chicago: American Hospital Association, 1995.

Buerhaus, P. I., and Staiger, D. O. "Managed Care and the Nurse Labor Market." *Journal of the American Medical Association,* 1996, *276*(18), 1487–1493.

Hess, J. D. "Education for Entry into Practice: An Ethical Perspective." *Journal of Professional Nursing,* Sept.-Oct. 1996, *12*(5), 289–296.

Institute of Medicine. *Nursing Staff in Hospitals and Nursing Homes: Is It Adequate?* G. S. Wunderlich, F. A. Sloan, and C. K. Davis (eds.). Washington, D.C.: National Academy Press, 1996.

Joint Commission on Accreditation of Healthcare Organizations. *1996 Comprehensive Accreditation Manual for Hospitals: Standards, Scoring Guidelines, Aggregation Rules, Decision Rules.* Oakbrook Terrace, Ill.: Joint Commission on the Accreditation of Healthcare Organizations, 1996.

Keegan, A. J. "Hospitals Become Cost Centers in Managed Care Scenario." *Healthcare Financial Management,* Aug. 1994.

Koerner, J. "Differentiated Practice: The Evolution of Professional Nursing." *Journal of Professional Nursing,* 1992, *8*, 335–341.

Lawrenz & Associates, Inc. Unpublished report. Princeton, N.J.: Lawrenz & Associates, Inc., 1994.

Moses, E. B. *The Registered Nurse Population: Findings from the National Sample Survey of Registered Nurses, March 1992.* Rockville, Md.: Division of Nursing, U.S. Bureau of Health Professions, Health Resources and Services Administration, Public Health Service, U.S. Department of Health and Human Services, 1994.

Moses, E. B. *The Registered Nurse Population: Findings from the National Sample Survey of Registered Nurses, March 1996.* Rockville, Md.: Division of Nursing, U.S. Bureau of Health Professions, Health Resources and Services Administration, Public Health Service, U.S. Department of Health and Human Services, 1997.

National Advisory Council on Nursing Education and Practice. *Report to the Secretary of Health and Human Services on the Basic Registered Nurse Workforce.* Washington, D.C.: U.S. Department of Health and Human Services, 1996.

National Commission on Nursing Implementation Project. "Nursing Vital Signs." *Shaping the Profession for the 1990s.*: Battle Creek, Mich.: W. K. Kellogg Foundation, Mar. 1990.

National League for Nursing. *Nursing Datasource 1995.* Pub. no. 19–6649. New York: NLN Press, 1995.

Pew Health Professions Commission. *Critical Challenges: Revitalizing the Health Professions for the Twenty-First Century.* San Francisco: UCSF Center for the Health Professions, 1995.

Primm, P. L. "Differentiated Practice for ADN-BSN Prepared Nurses." *Journal of Professional Nursing,* July-Aug. 1987, pp. 218–225.

Spetz, J. E. *Nursing Staff Trends in California Hospitals: 1977 Through 1995.* San Francisco: Public Policy Institute of California, Oct. 1996.

Stilwell, B. "Nursing Practice in Today's World." Background paper, World Health Organization Expert Committee on Nursing Practice. Geneva: World Health Organization, 1995, p. 6.

CHAPTER SIX

Nurses in Long-Term Care Facilities in the United States

Charlene Harrington

The aging of the U.S. population is one of the major forces shaping future demand for health services, especially long-term care. The cost containment pressures articulated in Chapter Five are compounding the trend toward delivery of more services in long-term care settings. However, as Harrington notes in this chapter, the rise in demand for long-term care does not necessarily signal increased employment opportunities for RNs. States are more carefully limiting the use of Medicaid dollars for nursing home support, and developing home- and community-based alternatives to nursing home admission. The industry is predominantly proprietary, a characteristic which has led to pressure to hold down wages, and use less-well-trained staff. Although there have been significant federal efforts to address historical concerns about the quality of long-term care, this part of the health care system continues to exhibit uneven quality. One measure proven to improve quality has been to increase RN staffing levels in these facilities. However, this strategy has yet to be implemented widely due to cost considerations.

Nursing facilities are an important component of the health care industry. This chapter examines the demand and supply for nursing facilities, the complex factors that influence the nursing home market, and their implications for RN employment in nursing facilities. In spite of the increased demand for long-term care services, the supply of nursing facilities is somewhat constrained because of economic and regulatory controls, including state certificate of need and state Medicaid reimbursement policies. The dominance of proprietary and chain-operated facilities and the orientation toward maximizing investor profits encourages facilities to restrict staffing levels and operating expenses.

Although some facilities are known to provide exceptional care, the quality of care varies widely. Despite federal and state regulatory efforts, quality continues to be problematic. Quality problems are closely associated with historically low registered nurse staffing levels in nursing facilities. Research shows that quality of nursing facility care could be improved by increasing the number of registered nurses and overall staffing levels. The redeployment of hospital nurses into nursing facilities could greatly enhance the quality of care and the image of the nursing home industry. Unfortunately, the current political and economic climate limits the feasibility of increasing nurse staffing levels as a means of improving the care for nursing home residents. These market factors will influence the number of nurses working in nursing homes in the future and their level of education.

NURSING FACILITY MARKET

Nursing home expenditures increased 8 percent between 1994 and 1995, and nursing home services accounted for approximately $80 billion or 8 percent of the total health care expenditures in the United States in 1995 (Burner and Waldo, 1995). Government comprises the largest payer of nursing home care. The Medicaid program paid for an estimated 49.7 percent of all the nation's nursing home expenditures in 1995 according to the Health Care Financing Administration (HCFA) actuaries. Medicare paid 11.8 percent and other government sources paid 2 percent of the total costs (Burner and Waldo, 1995). An estimated 32 percent was paid for directly out of pocket by consumers, 2.5 percent by private insurance, and 2 percent by other private sources.

Medicaid nursing home days of care account for a major proportion of all patient days (estimated at 74 percent in 1993 by HCIA and Arthur Andersen, 1995). Although Medicare benefits have been broadened considerably since 1989, Medicare coverage for long-term care continues to be limited to up to one hundred days for skilled nursing facility care after hospitalization. Those who need long-term care beyond Medicare must either pay for nursing home care directly out of pocket or spend down their resources to become eligible for Medicaid coverage for nursing home care. Because long-term nursing home care costs between $30,000 and $50,000 per year, many individuals are forced to spend their resources to become eligible for Medicaid (Short, Kemper, Cornelius, and Walden, 1992). The result is that the financing of the nursing home industry is distinctively different from hospital and physician services, which are primarily paid for by Medicare and private insurance.

Most nursing facilities prefer private-paying clients because facilities can generally charge private-paying residents higher daily rates than Medicaid will pay (Buchanan, Madel, and Persons, 1991). Private patient payment rates for nursing home care were 20 percent per day higher than Medicaid rates in 1987. Medicare reimbursement rates are also generally higher than Medicaid rates, so Medicare posthospital patients are sought after by facilities.

Most facilities that are certified for Medicare patients have a unit to provide care exclusively to such patients or specialize in caring for them, because these patients require additional resources and expertise. Some nursing homes, especially those located in hospitals, have developed subacute units to provide a level of care between acute and skilled nursing care. There is little agreement about the definitions of subacute care, but Medicare is the primary payer for this level (Aaronson, Zinn, and Rosko, 1995). Subacute care is considered to be a major growth area for nursing facilities, which was estimated to be $3.4 billion in 1994 and expected to grow to $9.4 billion by the year 2000 (HCIA and Arthur Andersen, 1995). Such growth, however, is primarily a conversion of nursing facility beds from Medicaid to Medicare certified.

As enrollment of elderly persons in managed care plans has grown, some nursing homes have been developing managed care contracts for Medicare members. As noted in other chapters, managed care plans have consistently reduced the use of acute care services for the nonelderly population, and proponents believe it will yield similar reductions for the elderly (Luft, 1987; Greenfield and others, 1992). Hospital admission rates for the Medicare HMO population have been about the same as fee-for-services, but Medicare HMO members use fewer days of care than the fee-for-service population (Miller and Luft, 1994). The trend to less hospital care for the elderly shifts more care for them into the home or into long-term care facilities. Managed care contracts for Medicare-covered nursing facility services are considered attractive to nursing homes as new revenue sources because these contracts may pay higher reimbursement rates than Medicaid.

Nursing facilities tend to prefer the least sick patients (unless they receive higher rates for sicker patients under case-mix reimbursement) or those for whom they can provide the most cost-efficient care (Holahan and Cohen, 1987; Falcone, Bolda, and Leak, 1991; Kenney and Holahan, 1990). When nursing facilities are selective in their admission policies, access to care for those individuals with the greatest need may be limited. Where the supply of nursing home beds is limited, problems in gaining access to needed services may be exacerbated (Falcone, Bolda, and Leak, 1991; Kenney and Holahan, 1990).

FACTORS INCREASING DEMAND FOR NURSING HOME SERVICES

The demand for nursing home services is growing with the increasing numbers of individuals who are aged and chronically ill. In 1990, about thirty-two million Americans were age sixty-five and older; this is projected to increase to sixty-four million in 2030 (Zedlewski and McBride, 1992). The population age eighty-five and over is growing faster than other age groups and is projected to be almost six times greater in the year 2050 (U.S. Bureau of the Census, 1993).

As the population ages and develops chronic illnesses, the need for long-term care services, including nursing home services, increases. The total risk of becoming a nursing home patient after age sixty-five is 43 percent and peaks at age seventy-five to eighty (Murtaugh, Kemper, and Spillman, 1990). The number of elderly needing nursing home care is expected to increase from about 1.8 million in 1990 to 4.3–5.3 million in 2030, depending upon the projection assumptions (Zedlewski and McBride, 1992; Mendelson and Schwartz, 1993).

In addition, the degree of medical instability, impairment, and severity of illness in nursing home residents is increasing (Hing, 1989; Kanda and Mezey, 1991; Shaughnessy, Schlenker, and Kramer, 1990). Cost containment pressures are resulting in admission to nursing homes of persons with more complex health care needs. Medical technology formerly used only in the hospital is being transferred to nursing facilities. The use of intravenous feedings and medication, ventilators, oxygen, special prosthetic equipment and devices, and other high technologies has made nursing home care more difficult and challenging (Shaughnessy, Schlenker, and Kramer, 1990). Consequently, nursing home residents require greater professional nursing care and supervision, evaluation, and resources than in the past.

Several federal policy changes in the 1980s have contributed to increased demand for nursing home services. In 1983, congressional adoption of Medicare prospective payment systems (PPSs) for hospitals resulted in shortened hospital stays and increased numbers of referrals and admissions to nursing facilities (Guterman and others, 1988; Neu and Harrison, 1988). Medicare has covered up to one hundred days of skilled nursing home care after discharge from the hospital. The criteria for eligibility for nursing home care, however, were very strict until April 1988, when HCFA issued new Medicare guidelines to the fiscal intermediaries clarifying and expanding the eligibility criteria for nursing homes (U.S. House, 1990). These guidelines eliminated the need requirements for rehabilitation care and allowed special procedures (such as intravenous feedings) to qualify for Medicare coverage (1988 HCFA Transmittal letter). The elimination of the prior hospitalization requirement and the relaxation of the limits on the spell of illness requirements also liberalized Medicare nursing home benefits and expanded the total nursing home spending substantially (Aaronson, Zinn, and Rosko, 1995). In 1988, the Catastrophic Health Care legislation, though largely repealed, contributed to an increase in Medicaid program utilization and costs by establishing and maintaining a minimum level of asset and income protection for spouses when determining Medicaid nursing home eligibility (Letsch, Lazenby, Levit, and Cowan, 1992). These policy changes have all encouraged the demand for nursing home services.

FACTORS CONSTRAINING DEMAND FOR NURSING HOME SERVICES

Yet, simultaneously, other factors are constraining the rate of growth in demand for nursing home services. Some states have adopted policies to control Medicaid nursing home demand, including controls on Medicaid eligibility policies and preadmission screening programs to limit or target access to nursing home services (Ellwood and Burwell, 1990; Harrington and Curtis, 1996; Snow, 1995).

Probably more importantly, home- and community-based alternatives to, or substitutes for, nursing home care are expanding rapidly, which may reduce the demand for nursing home care. Federal Medicare policies that expanded coverage for home care services have increased utilization dramatically during the last five years. Chapter Eight provides a detailed discussion of the growth of the home care industry. Although no research has determined the impact of the growth of home and community care on nursing home services, there appears to be a relationship between the declining nursing home occupancy rates and the expansion of home and community services.

SUPPLY OF NURSING HOME SERVICES

The total number of licensed nursing facilities, including skilled nursing facilities (SNFs for Medicare patients), nursing facilities (NFs for Medicaid patients), and dually certified facilities (for Medicare and Medicaid), was 17,243 in 1994. These facilities (both freestanding and hospital-based) had 1,767,805 beds in 1994 (Harrington, Swan, Bedney, and Carrillo, 1996). In addition to these facilities was a total of 6,717 licensed intermediate care facilities for the mentally retarded (ICF-MR) with 138,100 beds in 1994. All states license some residential care (other than nursing facilities). Depending upon their laws, these included board and care, personal care, foster care, and assisted living facilities. In 1994 there were 41,483 licensed residential care facilities for the aged with 666,127 beds (Harrington, Swan, Bedney, and Carrillo, 1996). In addition, there were other board and care facility beds for persons with mental or developmental disabilities and children.

Examination of growth trends enhances understanding of the industry. The number of licensed nursing facilities increased by about 2 percent annually during the 1978–1994 period (DuNah, Harrington, Bedney, and Carrillo, 1995; Harrington, Swan, Bedney, and Carrillo, 1996). Based on past growth trends, future bed growth for nursing facilities can be expected to continue at 1 or 2 percent annually. The growth in beds for ICF-MR facilities was about 4 percent, and the growth in residential care beds for the aged was about 5 percent between 1993 and 1994 (Harrington and Curtis, 1996). Residential care facilities, however, generally provide no nursing services.

One key concern is whether the growth in beds is keeping pace with the aging of the population. Previous studies have shown that growth has failed to meet the demand in some areas (Nyman, 1988a; Bishop, 1988). The most recent data show that the average number of nursing facility beds dropped from 610 per 1,000 persons aged eighty-five and over in 1978 to 502 in 1994 (a 17.8 percent decline) (DuNah, Harrington, Bedney, and Carrillo, 1995). Thus, the number of beds in most states is failing to keep pace with the growth in the oldest old population.

A recent survey of state officials reported that some states may have an undersupply while many states reported an oversupply of nursing facility beds and declining occupancy rates (DuNah, Harrington, Bedney, and Carillo, 1995). The overall U.S. occupancy rate in nursing facilities was about 90 percent in 1994, slightly lower than in 1985. These rates vary significantly across the nation, with the highest rates occurring in the northeast and the lowest in the west. Thus, some areas and states especially in the northeast appear to have shortages of nursing home services and others may have an adequate or oversupply (DuNah, Harrington, Bedney, and Carrillo, 1995; Harrington, Swan, Nyman, and Carrillo, 1997). Areas with shortages are of concern because they may limit access for those in need of services.

IMPACT OF STATE REIMBURSEMENT POLICIES

State Medicaid programs have undertaken a number of policy initiatives to control supply and reduce spending on nursing home care. This trend began in the early 1980s, when cuts in federal Medicaid spending became standard features of the budget process (Bishop, 1988). The most important policy affecting the supply of long-term care beds is the state certificate of need (CON) program.

The health planning and CON program established in 1974 (P.L. 94–641) gave states considerable authority and discretion to plan and control the capital expenditures for nursing facilities and other health facilities. The effectiveness of CON policies in controlling bed supply were widely debated, and the policies were opposed by many nursing homes. These controversies resulted in the federal repeal of the program in 1986 (Kosciesza, 1987). Even after the federal repeal of the program, forty states continued to use CON or moratoria policies to regulate the growth in nursing facilities in 1994 (Harrington, Swan, Nyman, and Carrillo, 1997). CON and moratoria policies for nursing facilities have been found to be associated with lower growth in bed ratios and higher occupancy rates (Harrington, Swan, Nyman, and Carrillo, 1997) and with lower costs to the Medicaid program (Harrington and Swan, 1987; Nyman, 1988a). Thus, because of the cost pressures on states, we can expect most states to continue their efforts to limit the supply of nursing home beds.

The second major policy that has constrained the growth in nursing home supply is state Medicaid reimbursement policy. States have considerable discretion in developing Medicaid reimbursement methods and rates. Many state Medicaid programs have attempted to control the growth in nursing home reimbursement rates (Swan, Harrington, and Grant, 1993; Holahan and Cohen, 1987; Bishop, 1988; Nyman, 1988a; Holahan, Rowland, Feder, and Heslam, 1993). In 1994, the average Medicaid rate across states was $80.79 per day, which was about 5.3 percent higher than for 1993 (Swan, DeWit, and Harrington, 1995). The national mean Consumer Price Index (CPI) adjusted rate in 1994 showed only a 1.4 percent increase over 1993. Overall average Medicaid reimbursement rates have increased only a total of 4.8 percent over inflation since 1990 (Swan, DeWit, and Harrington, 1995). Medicaid nursing home reimbursement rates vary widely across states in response to differences in methodologies but have been generally effective in controlling rate increases. The low growth in rates tends to suppress the overall growth in nursing home beds but also has a constraining effect on increases in nursing personnel.

Since 1980, there has been a pronounced shift away from retrospective reimbursement to prospective facility-specific methods or combination or adjusted systems (Swan, Harrington, and Grant, 1993; Swan, DeWit, and Harrington, 1995). Prospective reimbursement systems tend to lower Medicaid costs more than retrospective systems (Buchanan, Madel, and Persons, 1991; Swan, Harrington, and Grant, 1993; Swan, DeWit, and Harrington, 1995; Coburn, Fortinsky, McGuire, and McDonald, 1993). There also has been a substantial increase in numbers of states with case-mix reimbursement (nineteen case-mix states in 1993). By 1996, about half of all state Medicaid programs will be using case-mix reimbursement (Swan, DeWit, and Harrington, 1995).

OWNERSHIP STRUCTURE AND PROFITS

Nursing facility staffing levels, wages, and benefits have been low primarily because of the quest for profits in the nursing home industry. The majority of nursing facilities are proprietary, and facilities are increasingly owned by investors. Of the total certified nursing facilities, 66 percent were reported as proprietary, 27 percent were nonprofit, and 7 percent were government owned in 1995 (Harrington, Carrillo, Thollaug, and Summers, 1996). Although facilities can be classified by ownership, corporate goals differ within these ownership categories. Although nonprofit facilities generally have charitable goals, some may seek to maximize revenues in order to compete with proprietary facilities. The latter generally are oriented toward maximizing profits. These facilities make profits by reducing operating costs.

The trend toward consolidation of the health care industry, identified in Chapter One, is clearly evident among nursing facilities. In 1995, federal reports showed that about 51 percent of certified facilities were chain facilities (Harrington, Carrillo, Thollaug, and Summers, 1996). The largest twenty chains operated 18 percent of the total beds in the United States (HCIA and Arthur Anderson, 1994). The merger and acquisition activity has been high, with twenty-three of the twenty-five largest nursing home chains involved in acquisitions during 1993. In 1994, the merger and acquisition activity was reported at $60 billion (HCIA and Arthur Anderson, 1995). In addition, sixteen nursing home companies have become public in the past two years, which gives these companies new sources of capital for growth and acquisitions.

The health care industry, including the nursing home corporations, ranked first out of twenty-one industry groups for its five-year return on equity. The total profit margin for the free-standing nursing home industry (calculated as the difference between total net revenue and total expenses divided by total net revenues reported from facility cost reports) was reported at 6 percent for 1993 (HCIA and Arthur Anderson, 1995). Profit margins were higher in investor-owned and system-affiliated facilities than in other types, and higher in medium-sized facilities than in small ones.

QUALITY OF NURSING HOME CARE PROBLEMS

The quality of care provided in nursing facilities has long been a matter of great concern to consumers, health care professionals, and policymakers. The Institute of Medicine's Committee on Nursing Home Regulation (1986) reported widespread quality of care problems. The problems were confirmed by the U.S. General Accounting Office (1987) and the U.S. Senate (1986), which found that many of the nation's nursing facilities were not meeting minimum requirements for maintaining residents' health and safety. These continuing problems were described again by the Institute of Medicine Committee on the Adequacy of Nurse Staffing in Hospitals and Nursing Homes (1996).

Numerous studies have identified many negative outcomes in nursing facilities (Zinn, Aaronson, and Rosko, 1993a, 1993b). These include urinary incontinence, falls, weight loss, and infectious disease (Libow and Starer, 1989). Declines in physical functioning that could have been prevented are also important negative outcomes (Linn, Gurel, and Linn, 1977). Mortality rates or hospital readmission rates are simple outcome measures that are commonly used (Spector and Takada, 1991). Other common negative outcomes include accidents, behavioral and emotional problems, cognitive problems, psychotropic drug reactions, decubitus ulcers, and others (Zinn, 1993a; Zinn, Aaronson, and Rosko, 1993a, 1993b).

A number of clinical practices have been associated with poor patient outcomes. Urethral catheterization may place residents at greater risk for urinary infection and hospitalization or other complications such as bladder and renal stones, abscesses, and renal failure (Ouslander and Kane, 1984; Ribiero and Smith, 1985). The use of physical restraints is a common practice and continues to be a problem. Restraints have been under criticism because their use may cause decreased muscle tone and increased likelihood of falls, incontinence, pressure ulcers, depression, confusion, and mental deterioration (Evans and Strumpf, 1989; Phillips, Hawes, and Fries, 1993). Phillips, Hawes, and Fries concluded that providing a restraint-free environment is less costly and can improve the quality of care and quality of life for residents. Tube feedings also increase the risk of complications, including lung infections, aspiration, misplacement of the tube, and pain (Libow and Starer, 1989). The improper use of psychotrophic drugs has been identified as a common problem in nursing facilities in numerous studies (Harrington, Tompkins, Curtis, and Grant, 1992). Recent Senate hearings focused on the problems associated with the misuse and inappropriate use of chemical restraints, which the regulations established under Omnibus Budget Reconciliation Act (OBRA) of 1990 were designed to reduce (U.S. Senate, 1991).

Despite efforts to improve the quality of care in nursing homes, state surveyors continue to find problems. In order to participate in the Medicare or Medicaid programs, long-term care facilities are required to meet federal certification requirements established by HCFA (42 CFR Part 843) under the Social Security Act. Skilled nursing facilities (SNFs) are regulated under the Medicare statute (Title 18), nursing facilities (NFs) under the Medicaid statute (Title 19), and dually certified facilities under both the Medicare and Medicaid statutes. State survey agencies are authorized to determine whether SNFs and NFs meet the federal requirements. Surveyors conduct on-site inspections to observe care, review records, and determine compliance. These surveys are used as the basis for entering into, denying, or terminating a provider agreement with the facility. Table 6.1 presents the findings of care deficiencies in nursing facility surveys across the states in 1991 and 1995. The frequency of these deficiencies shows that quality problems continue to exist in many nursing facilities. Probably no other type of health care organization has been demonstrated to have so many quality of care problems as nursing facilities. This demonstrates the need for continued research and the development of public policies that could improve both the process and outcomes of care.

Table 6.1. Nursing Facility Deficiencies in 1991 and 1995.

Deficiency	Percent of Facilities	
	1991	1995*
Comprehensive assessments	27	31
Comprehensive care plans	32	25
Food sanitation	29	24
Accident environment	19	18
Housekeeping	20	18
Maintain dignity	20	16
Physical restraint	21	15
Accommodate needs	19	15
Infection control	20	14
Pressure sores	20	14

*Data for only the first six months of 1995

Source: Harrington, Carrillo, Thollaug, and Summers, 1996

The OBRA 1987 Nursing Home Reform legislation, implemented by Health Care Financing Administration regulations in October 1990, mandated a number of changes. First, it eliminated the priority hierarchy of conditions, standards, and elements that were in the prior regulations. Second, it mandated comprehensive assessments of all nursing home residents using the new Minimum Data Set (MDS) forms (Morris and others, 1990) Third, more specific requirements for nursing, medical, and psychosocial services were designed to ensure that residents attain and maintain the highest practicable mental and physical functional status (Zimmerman, 1990).

The Nursing Home Resident Assessment System was designed to improve the resident assessment of specific problem areas and to guide the care planning process (Morris and others, 1990). Nursing facilities must complete the MDS forms for each resident within fourteen days of admission and at least annually in order to assess the functional, cognitive, and affective levels of residents and must use the assessment in the care planning process. The MDS includes the following fifteen domains: cognitive patterns, communication/hearing patterns, vision patterns, physical functioning and structural problems, continence, psychosocial well-being, mood and behavior patterns, activity pursuit patterns, disease diagnoses, health conditions, oral/nutritional status, oral/dental status, skin condition, medication use, and special treatments and procedures (Morris and others, 1990). The resident assessments must be completed by a multidisciplinary team in each facility and signed by a registered nurse. Currently, Zimmerman and others (1995) are developing quality indicators (QIs) that use the MDS in a study funded by HCFA. The QIs for individual residents and for facilities are compared to national norms, taking into account predisposing factors and case-mix factors related to each QI.

NURSING HOME STAFFING STANDARDS

Because there has consistently been a correlation between higher nurse staffing and better quality of care in nursing facilities, the Institute of Medicine Committee on Nursing Home Regulation (1986) recommended that nurse staffing standards be increased to improve the overall quality of nursing care. Following this recommendation, Congress increased the minimum standards for nursing home staffing in OBRA 1987. Implemented in the 1990 Medicare and Medicaid regulations for SNFs and NFs, this legislation requires an RN director of nursing, an RN on duty for eight hours a day seven days a week, and a licensed nurse (RN, LPN or LVN) on duty around the clock (U.S. Department of Health and Human Services, 1991). OBRA 1987 also requires that nursing assistants receive minimum training (seventy-five hours) and be tested for competency. In addition, "sufficient" nursing staff is required to provide nursing and related services to attain or maintain the highest practicable level of physical, mental, and psychosocial well-being of each resident.

Both Medicare and Medicaid staffing regulations require nursing homes to base staffing patterns on the actual care needs of residents. Medicare has traditionally required higher staffing levels because Medicare beneficiaries admitted to nursing facilities had more extensive care needs than their Medicaid counterparts. Many Medicare certified beds are in acute care facilities where staffing levels have been higher than in freestanding facilities. Medicare payment rates are substantially higher than Medicaid rates to take these higher resident care and resource needs into account (Dor, 1989).

The OBRA 1987 legislation allowed for waivers to the minimal nursing facility staffing requirements in areas where it may be difficult to hire registered nurses. Staffing waivers for Medicaid-only certified facilities (Title 19) can be granted by states, whereas staffing waivers for Medicare/Medicaid (Title 18/19 facilities) or Medicare-only certified facilities (Title 18) must be granted by HCFA. The law allows both the twenty-four hour licensed nursing coverage requirements and the eight hours of RN coverage seven days a week to be waived by state Medicaid programs, but Medicare facilities are only allowed to have waivers for the eight hours of RN coverage for two out of seven days a week. Recent data from HCFA suggest that the number of waivers for staffing is declining (Institute of Medicine, 1996). It is expected that the number of waivers will continue to decline as the availability of RNs improves with recent layoffs of hospital nurses.

STAFFING LEVELS

Detailed staffing data for certified nursing facilities are available from the federal On-Line Survey Certification and Reporting System (OSCAR). These reports show that in 1991 the average ratio of RNs was 0.4 hours (twenty-four minutes) per resident day, LPN-LVNs 0.6 hours (thirty-six minutes), and nursing assistants 2.0 hours (120 minutes), for a total of 3.0 nursing hours per resident day in about 15,500 nursing facilities in the United States (Harrington, Carrillo, Thollaug, and Summers, 1996). Table 6.2 displays these data. (This is calculated by dividing the total average nursing homes per day by the total average number of nursing residents per day.) By 1995, U.S. nursing facilities were reporting 0.5 RN hours per resident (30 minutes), 0.7 LVN-LPN hours, and 2.1 nursing assistant hours for a total of 3.3 hours per resident day (Harrington, Swan, Bedney, and Carrillo, 1996). Thus, there was only a small increase in nursing staff hours over the five-year period.

Staffing levels for Medicare-only certified facilities were substantially higher but represented only about 1,600 facilities out of the about 15,500 reporting. For Medicare-only facilities, the RN hours per resident day increased from 1.0 (sixty minutes) in 1991 to 1.7 in 1995 (102 minutes). The LPN-LVN hours per resident day increased from 1.2 in 1991 to 1.5 in 1995, and the nursing assistant hours per resident day increased from 2.4 to 3.0 hours over the period (Harrington, Carrillo, Thollaug, and Summers, 1996). Thus, staffing levels for all categories increased somewhat over the five-year period.

Table 6.2. Nursing Staffing Levels for Certified Nursing Facilities, 1991 and 1995.

	1991	1995*
Medicaid Only &		
Medicare/Medicaid ($n = 13, 600$)		
RN hours per resident day	0.3	0.4
LVN/LPN hours per resident day	0.6	0.6
Aide hours per resident day	2.0	2.0
Total nurse hours	2.9	3.0
Medicare-Only Facilities ($n = 1,700$)		
RN hours per resident day	1.0	1.7
LVN/LPN hours per resident day	1.2	1.5
Aide hours per resident day	2.4	3.0
Total nurse hours	4.4	5.6

*Data for only the first six months of 1995

Source: Harrington, Carrillo, Thollaug, and Summers, 1996

However, this apparent increase may be misleading. The ratios reported do not take into account vacation and sick time estimates and other factors in staffing. Moreover, and more importantly, nursing staff are not evenly distributed over twenty-four hours. Most health facilities have fewer staff on evening and night shifts because there are somewhat fewer care activities than during the day. Staffing is usually lower on holidays and weekends in terms of both licensed personnel ratios and total numbers of staff. Thus, a higher average staffing ratio may not reflect a uniform increase in nurse staffing throughout the day and year.

Zinn also found (1993b) that nursing facilities adjust staffing and care practices to local market conditions as would be expected. Her study of 14,000 nursing facilities in 1987 found that nursing facilities respond to local economic factors. In areas where RN wages were higher, nursing facilities employed more nonprofessional nursing staff. Thus, nursing facilities have economic incentives to hire fewer nursing personnel, especially in high-cost market areas.

STAFFING LEVELS AND QUALITY OF CARE

Not surprisingly, higher RN staffing levels in nursing facilities have been associated with higher quality of care. One of the first studies to document this relationship found that homes with more RN hours per resident were associated with lower mortality rates, improved physical health, and a higher rate of discharge home (Linn, Gurel, and Linn, 1977). Nyman (1988b) found that higher nursing hours per resident were significantly and positively associated with three of eight quality measures in Iowa nursing facilities. Nyman, Breaker, and Link (1990) found that the quality of life in a nursing home was associated with the general staffing level. More specifically, this study found that facilities with a higher percentage of nurse supervisory hours were more efficient and that the percentage of administrator hours was not related to efficiency. Nyman (1988b) showed that quality in nursing facilities is not associated with cost and that quality can be improved.

Gustafson, Sainfort, Van Konigsveld, and Zimmerman (1990) found a significant correlation between staffing and six measures of quality incorporated into the Quality Assurance Indicator index. Munroe's study (1990) of skilled nursing facilities found a positive relationship between nursing home quality (as measured by the number of health-related deficiencies) and the number of RN and LVN nursing hours provided. Spector and Takada (1991), in a study of 2,500 nursing home residents in eighty nursing facilities in Rhode Island, found that low staffing in homes with very dependent residents was associated with reduced likelihood of improvement. High urinary catheter use, low rates of skin care, and low resident participation rates in organized activities were all associated with poor resident outcomes. High RN turnover was also associated with decreased likelihood of functional improvement.

Zinn (1993b) conducted a study using data from 14,000 nursing facilities and found that higher RN wages were associated with lower ratios of RN staff to residents employed by nursing facilities. Fewer RNs were associated with higher use of urinary catheters, physical restraints, tube feedings, and not toileting residents. These negative resident conditions were also more likely to be associated with greater case-mix severity, lower private-pay rates in a county, higher proprietary ownership, and less concentration of the nursing home market. Another recent study of nursing facilities using the 1987 data from 449 freestanding nursing facilities in Pennsylvania found that nonprofit nursing facilities provided significantly higher quality of care to Medicaid beneficiaries and to self-pay residents than for-profit facilities, controlling for case mix (Aaronson, Zinn, and Rosko, 1994). Nonprofit facilities also had higher staffing levels.

As noted, reductions in the levels of RN staffing are a growing concern for quality of care because of recent controls on Medicaid reimbursement and prospective payment for hospitals and subsequent reductions in staffing levels (Kanda and Mezey, 1991). The preponderance of evidence from a number of studies with different types of quality measures has shown a positive relationship between higher nursing staffing and quality of nursing home care (Institute of Medicine, 1996). Thus, it can be concluded that lower staffing levels are related to poor process and outcome measures of nursing facility quality.

This low level of registered-nurse staffing in nursing facilities prompted a recent committee at the Institute of Medicine (1996) to recommend adding more staffing in nursing facilities in the report *Nursing Staff in Hospitals and Nursing Homes: Is It Adequate?* Specifically, the report recommended beginning by requiring facilities to have twenty-four-hour (rather than eight-hour) per day RN staffing at a minimum in all nursing facilities. Beyond the minimum levels, facilities are expected to ensure adequate staffing to meet the needs of nursing facility residents.

APPROPRIATE NURSE STAFFING STANDARDS

A strong relationship between resident characteristics, nurse staffing time requirements, and nursing costs in nursing facilities has been shown in several studies (Arling, Nordquist, Brant, and Capitman, 1987; Fries and Cooney, 1985; Schneider and others, 1988; Fries and others, 1994). Many nursing experts and consumer groups have argued that the current minimum HCFA nursing standards are too low and should be increased (Mezey, Lynaugh, and Cartier, 1989). Moreover, consumers suggest that the OBRA requirement for "sufficient staff" does not provide clear direction to nursing facilities and adequate protection of residents (National Citizens Coalition for Nursing Home Reform, 1994). However, experts have yet to reach a consensus as to how nurse staffing standards should be improved.

In 1987, a panel of nurse experts from the Executive Committee of the Council on Nursing Administration of the American Nurses' Association proposed a minimum staffing approach for nursing facilities based on expert opinion (Turner, 1987). They recommended that direct caregivers ratios (including RNs, LVNs, and NAs) should be established at one to eight during the day, one to ten in the evening, and one to fifteen at night. Another approach is to use the current staffing patterns in Medicare-certified facilities as a minimum standard for all facilities.

The national Casemix Demonstration Project has conducted two studies of staffing requirements for different case-mix levels (Feldman, 1996; Fries and others, 1994). These data can be used as guidelines for minimum staffing standards depending on the characteristics of residents in each facility. HCFA should expand and detail its minimum standards for nursing facilities and develop guidelines for state survey agency inspectors to determine whether or not facilities are complying with the minimum staffing levels.

POOR NURSING COMPENSATION AND ITS CONSEQUENCES

One major reason that RN staffing in nursing homes is often inadequate is the low salaries and benefits relative to what nurses earn in other settings, such as hospitals. The overall average annual earnings of registered nurses employed full-time in nursing facilities was $37,458 in 1996. Average staff nurses in nursing facilities had annual earnings 14 percent below average hospital staff nurses (Moses, 1997). This was especially low, considering that RNs working in nursing facilities were more likely to be administrators (19 percent) than were nurses in hospitals (2 percent) (Moses, 1997). In fact, the average salary of nursing home nurses was lower than salaries in any other setting except student health care services (Moses, 1997).

Salary levels were lower in investor-owned facilities and system-affiliated facilities and higher in nonprofit facilities. They were also lower in smaller facilities (HCIA and Arthur Anderson, 1994). The fact that many nursing facilities do not provide their employees with health benefits is also a problem. Recently, the American Health Care Association (1994) estimated that if mandatory national health insurance were adopted by Congress, nursing facilities costs passed on to Medicaid would increase by $1 billion and costs to Medicare would increase by $100 million.

Poor nursing home compensation encourages nurses to seek employment in other health care settings or outside the industry in better working environments.

The traditionally high employee turnover rates in some facilities are directly related to low salaries and benefits (Harrington, 1990). Nursing home nurses have had higher turnover rates than hospital nurses. Only 81.2 percent of nursing home RNs reported working in a nursing home in the previous year compared with 92.2 percent for hospital nurses (Moses, 1997). Munroe (1990) found RN turnover rates of over 100 percent in California nursing facilities in 1986, which were associated with poor quality (in terms of the number of deficiencies identified). Where there is an adequate supply of nursing personnel, some nursing facilities may encourage high turnover rates as a means of keeping average wage rates low (Harrington, 1990).

Compensation for nursing home nurses will continue to be an issue as hospitals downsize. As noted throughout this book and in the report of the Institute of Medicine's Committee on the Adequacy of Nurse Staffing in Hospitals and Nursing Homes (1996), the downsizing and restructuring of hospitals can be expected to continue in the future due to the dramatic growth in managed care, which reduces the need for hospital care. This reduction may increase the number of nurses available to work in nursing homes and other settings outside of hospitals. The competition among RNs for employment may stabilize nursing home staffing and reduce the turnover rates. But unless nursing home staffing ratios, wages, and benefits are increased to levels comparable to the rest of the health industry, nursing homes will continue to be a less desirable workplace for nurses than other health settings.

INADEQUATE EDUCATIONAL TRAINING

There are many concerns about the adequacy of the education and training of nursing home personnel. The 1996 National Sample Survey of Registered Nurses estimated that 170,856 RNs (8.1 percent of RNs employed in nursing) work in nursing facilities or extended care facilities (Moses, 1997). RNs working in nursing facilities on average were more likely to have a lower level of education than nurses working in hospitals. More RNs working in nursing homes were educated at the diploma level (30.4 percent) compared with those working in hospitals (22.3 percent) (Moses, 1997). RNs in nursing homes were less likely to have a baccalaureate or master's degree than RNs in other settings. These lower education levels may be related to the low salaries and benefits in nursing facilities. Nurses with higher education levels can be expected to seek employment in hospitals and other settings where they can receive higher wages and benefits. In other situations, facilities may employ nurses with less education as a means of keeping salaries low.

Another concern is the inadequate training that most nursing home personnel have had in geriatrics and gerontological nursing. A specialty area has developed in gerontological nursing with a strong knowledge base that argues for the necessity of geriatric training to improve the quality of care for the aged (Matteson and McConnell, 1988). The increased complexity of care required for nursing home residents (Shaughnessy, Schlenker, and Kramer, 1990) makes the need for specialty training even greater. Directors of nursing and supervisors in nursing facilities need advanced training in gerontology, but few have it.

A number of nursing facilities have developed important initiatives to improve the quality of care by improving training and adding specially trained nursing staff. The National Institute on Aging and the Robert Wood Johnson (RWJ) Foundation both initiated teaching nursing home programs to improve quality of care during the 1980s. The RWJ project was a five-year program in twelve nursing facilities, ending in 1987, that added geriatric and geropsychiatric nurse practitioners and clinicians to nursing facilities in collaboration with schools of nursing. This project was found to reduce hospitalization rates, bowel incontinence, restraint use, and urinary incontinence and to improve care (Mezey, Lynaugh, and Cartier, 1989; Mezey and Lynaugh, 1991). The success of these programs has been documented in a series of articles and books (Shaughnessy and Kramer, 1989; Mezey, Lynaugh, and Cartier, 1989).

Kane and others (1988), in a study of geriatric nurse practitioners employed in thirty nursing facilities, found that in spite of the difficulties in developing new roles for geriatric nurse practitioners, two-thirds of the facilities were enthusiastic about the program. Kane and others (1989), using data from the same study, found modest improvements in the process of care with the addition of geriatric nurse practitioners, but no consistent changes in health outcomes. Buchanan and others (1990), also using data from the same study, found that the employment of geriatric nurse practitioners does not adversely affect nursing home costs or profits, and that geriatric nurse practitioners do reduce the use of hospital services. Geriatric nurse practitioners can provide special geriatric care to address common problems of nursing home residents and can provide geriatric training for staff.

These studies used geriatric nurse practitioners as consultants to the facilities, not in primary care roles for patient management. Using geriatric nurse practitioners in primary care roles as substitutes for physician care may have a greater beneficial effect than using geriatric nurse practitioners as specialty nursing employees (Buchanan and others, 1990).

Some experts in nursing homes have concluded that nursing education is not preparing its new graduates adequately to assess the nursing home residents appropriately and develop sound care plans. One particular gap in training of nursing home nurses is reflected in the state survey (Table 6.1), which found the largest number of deficiencies in nursing facilities that concerned failures to complete federally required comprehensive assessments and care plans. A recent study documented extensive problems in these areas. State survey agencies and nurses in a sample of nursing homes all reported that nurses receive poor training in the conduct of a comprehensive resident assessment and that the development of care plans for residents is poor (Harrington, Summers, Curtis, and Maynard, 1996). Because some nurses are having problems conducting the minimum resident assessments and developing adequate care plans, the resulting care for residents is often poor.

IMPROVING EDUCATION AND TRAINING

The education and training needs for registered nurses, licensed practical and vocational nurses, and nursing assistants in nursing homes are overwhelming (Institute of Medicine, 1996). As mentioned, many nurses have not had basic education in how to conduct comprehensive assessments and how to plan and implement care plans for nursing home residents, and many nursing programs provide little education on the aging process, gerontological nursing care, and care of nursing home residents (Bahr, 1991). The lack of training that nurses receive in the management and supervision of nursing assistants has also been cited as a major gap in the current educational preparation of nurses.

One way to improve the quality of nursing home care could be the employment of geriatric nursing specialists and practitioners to provide leadership in nursing homes and to oversee the provision of care to residents. This evidence led the IOM Committee on Nursing Staffing in Hospitals and Nursing Homes to recommend (1996) the expanded use of geriatric nurse specialists and practitioners in both leadership and direct care positions in nursing homes.

Other experts consider the training of nursing assistants in caring for nursing home residents to be seriously deficient (Burgio and Burgio, 1990). The IOM committee recommended new efforts for training nursing assistants in appropriate clinical care of the aged and disabled, occupational health and safety measures, culturally sensitive care, and appropriate management of conflict.

The nursing administration responsibilities in nursing homes are becoming increasingly complex. The need for improved nursing leadership within nursing homes is obvious considering all the problems identified with poor quality of care. The evidence suggests that most directors of nursing in nursing facilities are not academically prepared for their positions (Bahr, 1991). Few have specific education in aging, gerontological care, and management, and few have a bachelor's degree or advanced clinical training. These needs led the IOM committee to recommend that nursing facilities should place a higher weight on education when selecting new directors of nursing. The committee considered that a bachelor's degree in nursing with special training in management and gerontology should be the basic preparation for directors of nursing in nursing facilities.

POLITICAL BARRIERS

Several barriers exist to increasing the staffing, education, and training require-ments in nursing facilities. The first and most important one is economic. because government pays for over 63 percent of current nursing home expen-ditures (Burner and Waldo, 1995). Since OBRA 1987 was passed, selected con-gressional representatives have considered legislation that would increase staffing beyond the OBRA requirements, but such legislation has not had the political support to proceed. On the state level, the outlook is no better. Al-though states have the authority to increase their Medicaid payment rates as a means of increasing staffing standards, the economic problems facing the states with growing Medicaid budgets make it unlikely that states will initiate increases in nursing home staffing requirements.

A major barrier to increased staffing requirements is that nursing facilities have not always used state Medicaid rate increases to improve resident care. In the past, some Medicaid rate increases were not used to increase staffing and presumably were used by some facilities to improve profitability (Feder and Scanlon, 1989; Weissert and Musliner, 1992a, 1992b). Thus some officials are unwilling to support additional profit making. However, current Medicaid and Medicare reimbursement allocations could be used to redistribute existing pay-ments toward resident care.

Another problem is the historic opposition of the nursing home industry to regulation, which represents a major political obstacle to regulatory reform. Al-though the nursing home industry supports financial incentives for higher qual-ity, their opposition to further regulation stifles reform efforts. Consumer and professional organizations have not had the political power to counter the oppo-sition of the nursing home industry to new regulation in the current economic and political environment.

CONCLUSION

The nursing home market is being strained by a growing demand for services. The aging population and the greater acuity of illness and disability of individ-uals needing long-term care are placing new demands on providers of care.

Although a number of nursing home facilities in the United States have demon-strated that they can provide high-quality care even under the current economic constraints, the quality provided by nursing facilities varies and remains prob-lematic despite increased regulatory efforts. Direct patient care and nurse staffing are critical structural factors that affect both the process and the outcomes of care.

Quality of care could be improved not only by increasing nurse staffing levels but also by increasing training in gerontology and planning and management skills. Although inadequate nurse staffing levels have been shown to be a major factor in poor quality of nursing home care, nursing staffing levels in nursing facilities remain low compared to those of hospitals, particularly in proprietary nursing facilities. Low salaries and benefits contribute to quality of care problems and are associated with high staff turnover rates and low staff educational levels in nursing facilities.

Despite growing demand and widespread recognition that quality problems could be mitigated by increasing nurse staffing levels and enhancing the education of nursing home nurses, several factors, primarily economic, constrain opportunities for reform. Nursing home facilities are primarily private profit-making organizations that are increasingly part of multiorganizational systems and investor-owned corporations. Consequently, nursing facilities are oriented toward increasing profits. Reimbursement policies that allow facilities to make profits by lowering staffing levels and quality of care are problematic. Moreover, as most states have adopted Medicaid prospective payment systems and strict methods for controlling costs, major problems with access and quality have developed. Clearly, new and improved reimbursement approaches, such as Medicare's decision to eliminate return on equity payments, are needed that provide incentives to improve quality and staffing levels.

Although the regulation of nursing facility quality may have improved since the implementation of OBRA 1987, more stringent nurse staffing requirements are needed (Institute of Medicine, 1996). One problem with increasing staffing requirements is that the increased costs would fall primarily on the Medicaid and Medicare programs. Government officials have been reluctant to adopt new policies that would increase federal and state costs, even though such policies could be feasible if cost controls were placed on other components of nursing home costs. There is some evidence that limiting profits, administrative costs, and capital costs could achieve a savings that could shift funds to improve the quality of direct resident care.

The need for more highly trained nursing professionals in nursing homes is very apparent. However, it is unlikely that the industry will voluntarily increase the number of RNs and APNs without increased federal payment for such staff. This situation contrasts markedly with the ambulatory care and home care sectors, in which RN and APN employment is expanding (see Chapters Seven and Eight). The drive for increased profits and decreased government regulation makes the situation for nursing home residents very poor in the near future. Without great public outrage about the poor quality of care and without expanded federal funding for nursing homes, the poor nurse compensation and staffing situation can be expected to continue.

References

Aaronson, W. E., Zinn, J. S., and Rosko, M. D. "Do For-Profit and Not-for-Profit Nursing Homes Behave Differently?" *The Gerontologist*, 1994, *34*(6), 775–786.

Aaronson, W. E., Zinn, J. S., and Rosko, M. D. "Subacute Care, Medicare Benefits, and Nursing Home Behavior." *Medical Care Research and Review*, 1995, *52*(3), 364–388.

American Health Care Association. "Costs of an Employer Health Care Mandate." *Provider*, 1994, *20*(5), 8.

Arling, G., Nordquist, R. H., Brant, B. A., and Capitman, J. A. "Nursing Home Case Mix." *Medical Care*, 1987, *25*, 9–19.

Bahr, R. T. *Mechanisms of Quality in Long Term Care: Service and Clinical Outcomes.* Pub. No 41-2382. New York: National League for Nursing, 1991.

Bishop, C. E. "Competition in the Market for Nursing Home Care." *Journal of Health Politics, Policy and Law*, 1988, *13*(2), 341–361.

Buchanan, J. L., and others. "Assessing Cost Effects of Nursing-Home-Based Geriatric Nurse Practitioners." *Health Care Financing Review*, 1990, *11*(3), 67–78.

Buchanan, R. J., Madel, R. P., and Persons, D. "Medicaid Payment Policies for Nursing Home Care: A National Survey." *Health Care Financing Review*, 1991, *13*(1), 55–72.

Burgio, L. D., and Burgio, K. L. "Institutional Staff Training and Management: A Review of the Literature and a Model for Geriatric, Long-Term Care Facilities." *International Journal of Aging and Human Development*, 1990, *30*(4), 287–302.

Burner, S. T., and Waldo, D. R. "National Health Expenditure Projections, 1994–2005." *Health Care Financing Review*, 1995, *16*(4), 221–242.

Coburn, A. F., Fortinsky, R., McGuire, C., and McDonald, T. P. "Effect of Prospective Reimbursement on Nursing Home Costs." *Health Services Research*, 1993, *28*(1), 44–68.

Dor, A. "The Costs of Medicare Patients in Nursing Homes in the United States." *Journal of Health Economics*, 1989, *8*, 253–270.

DuNah, R., Harrington, C., Bedney, B., and Carrillo, H. "Variations and Trends in State Nursing Facility Capacity, 1978–93." *Health Care Financing Review*, 1995, *17*(1), 183–199.

Ellwood, M. R., and Burwell, B. "Access to Medicaid and Medicare by the Low-Income Disabled." *Health Care Financing Review*, 1990 Annual Supplement, pp. 133–148.

Evans, L., and Strumpf, N. "Tying Down the Elderly." *Journal of the American Geriatrics Society*, 1989, *37*, 65–74.

Falcone, D., Bolda, E., and Leak, S. "Waiting for Placement: An Exploratory Analysis of Determinants of Delayed Discharges of Elderly Patients." *Health Services Research*, 1991, *26*(3), 339–374.

Feder, J., and Scanlon, W. "Case-Mix Payment for Nursing Home Care: Lessons from Maryland." *Journal of Health Politics, Policy and Law*, 1989, *14*(3), 523–547.

Feldman, J. "Nursing Time Study." Paper presented at the National Care Mix Conference, San Antonio, Tex., Jan. 1996.

Fries, B. E., and Cooney, L. "Resources Utilization Groups: A Patient Classification System for Long-Term Care." *Health Care Financing Review,* 1985, *23*(2), 110–122.

Fries, B. E., and others. "Refining a Case-Mix Measure for Nursing Homes: Resources Utilization Groups (RUGS-III)." *Medical Care,* 1994, *32*(7), 668–685.

Greenfield, S., and others. "Variations in Resource Utilization Among Medical Specialties and Systems of Care: Results from the Medical Outcomes Study." *Journal of the American Medical Association,* 1992, *267*(12), 1624–1630.

Gustafson, D. H., Sainfort, F. C., Van Konigsveld, R., and Zimmerman, D. R. "The Quality Assessment Index (QAI) for Measuring Nursing Home Quality." *Health Services Research,* 1990, *25*(1), 97–127.

Guterman, S., and others. "The First 3 Years of Medicare Prospective Payment: An Overview." *Health Care Financing Review,* 1988, *9*(3), 67–77.

Harrington, C. "Wages and Benefits of Nursing Personnel in Nursing Homes: Correcting the Inequities." *Nursing Economic$,* 1990, *8*(6), 378–385.

Harrington, C., Carrillo, H., Thollaug, S., and Summers, P. *Nursing Facilities, Staffing, Residents, and Facility Deficiencies, 1991–95.* Report prepared for the Health Care Financing Administration. San Francisco: University of California, 1996.

Harrington, C., and Curtis, M. "State Variations in Trends in Preadmission Screening Programs." *Journal of Applied Gerontology,* 1996, *15*(4), 414–432.

Harrington, C., Summers, P., Curtis, M., and Maynard, R. *Study of the Accuracy of the Resident Assessment System in Nursing Homes.* Report prepared for the Health Care Financing Administration. San Francisco: University of California, 1996.

Harrington, C., and Swan, J. H. "The Impact of State Medicaid Nursing Home Policies on Utilization and Expenditures." *Inquiry,* 1987, *24,* 157–172.

Harrington, C., Swan, J. H., Bedney, B., and Carrillo, H. *1994 Long Term Care Program and Market Characteristics.* Prepared for the Department of Housing and Urban Development and the Health Care Financing Administration. San Francisco: University of California, 1996.

Harrington, C., Swan, J. H., Nyman, J. A., and Carrillo, H. "The Effect of Certificate of Need and Moratoria Policy on Change in Nursing Home Beds in the US." *Medical Care,* 1997, *35*(6), 574–588.

Harrington, C., Tompkins, C., Curtis, M., and Grant, L. "Psychotropic Drug Use in Long Term Care Facilities: A Review of the Literature." *The Gerontologist,* 1992, *32*(6), 822–833.

Harrington, C., and others. "State Regulation of the Supply of Long Term Care Providers." *Journal of Applied Gerontology,* 1997, *16*(9), 5–30.

HCIA and Arthur Andersen. *1994 Guide to the Nursing Home Industry.* Baltimore: HCIA, Inc., and Arthur Andersen & Company, 1994.

HCIA and Arthur Andersen. *1995 Guide to the Nursing Home Industry.* Baltimore: HCIA, Inc., and Arthur Andersen & Company, 1995.

Hing, E. *Effects of the Prospective Payment System on Nursing Homes.* DHHS Publication No. PHS–89–1759. Washington, D.C.: National Center for Health Statistics, 1989.

Holahan, J., and Cohen, J. "Nursing Home Reimbursement: Implications for Cost Containment, Access, and Quality." *Milbank Quarterly,* 1987, *65*(1), 112–147.

Holahan, J., Rowland, D., Feder, J., and Heslam, D. "Explaining the Recent Growth in Medicaid Spending." *Health Affairs,* Fall 1993, pp. 177–193.

Institute of Medicine, Committee on Nursing Home Regulation. "Introduction" and "Summary." In *Improving the Quality of Care in Nursing Homes.* Washington, D.C.: National Academy Press, 1986, pp. 1–44.

Institute of Medicine, Committee on the Adequacy of Nurse Staffing in Hospitals and Nursing Homes. *Nursing Staff in Hospitals and Nursing Homes: Is It Adequate?* G. S. Wunderlich, F. A. Sloan, C. K. Davis (eds.). Washington, D.C.: National Academy Press, 1996.

Kanda, K., and Mezey, M. "Registered Nurse Staffing in Pennsylvania Nursing Homes: Comparison Before and After Implementation of Medicare's Prospective Payment System." *The Gerontologist,* 1991, *31*(3), 318–324.

Kane, R. A., and others. "Geriatric Nurse Practitioners as Nursing Home Employees: Implementing the Role." *The Gerontologist,* 1988, *28*(4), 469–477.

Kane, R. L., and others. "Effect of a Geriatric Nurse Practitioner on the Process and Outcomes of Nursing Home Care." *American Journal of Public Health,* 1989, *79*(9), 1271–1277.

Kenney, G., and Holahan, J. "The Nursing Home Market and Hospital Discharge Delays." *Inquiry,* 1990, *27*, 73–85.

Kosciesza, I. "What's Ahead in the Post-Health Planning Era." *Health Policy Week Special Report,* June 1, 1987, pp. 1–5.

Letsch, S. W., Lazenby, H. C., Levit, L. R., and Cowan, C. A. "National Health Expenditures, 1991." *Health Care Financing Review,* 1992, *14*(2), 1–30.

Libow, L., and Starer, P. "Care of the Nursing Home Patient." *New England Journal of Medicine,* 1989, *321*, 93–96.

Linn, M., Gurel, L., and Linn, B. A. "Patient Outcome as a Measure of Quality of Nursing Home Care." *American Journal of Public Health,* 1977, *67*, 337–344.

Luft, H. *Health Maintenance Organizations: Dimension of Performance.* New Brunswick, Conn.: Transition Books, 1987.

Matteson, M., and McConnell, E. S. *Gerontological Nursing.* Philadelphia: Saunders, 1988.

Mendelson, D. N., and Schwartz, W. B. "The Effects of Aging and Population Growth on Health Care Costs." *Health Affairs,* 1993, *12*(1), 119–125.

Mezey, M. D., and Lynaugh, J. E. "Teaching Nursing Home Program: A Lesson in Quality." *Geriatric Nursing,* Mar.-Apr. 1991, pp. 76–77.

Mezey, M. D., Lynaugh, J. E., and Cartier, M. M. (eds.). *Nursing Homes and Care: Lessons from Teaching Nursing Homes.* New York: Springer, 1989.

Miller, R. H., and Luft, H. S. "Managed Care Plan Performance Since 1980: A Literature Analysis." *Journal of the American Medical Association,* 1994, *271*(10), 1512–1519.

Morris, J., and others. "Designing the National Resident Assessment Instrument for Nursing Homes." *The Gerontologist,* 1990, *30*(3), 293–307.

Moses, E. B. *The Registered Nurse Population: Findings from the National Sample Survey of Registered Nurses, March 1992.* Rockville, Md.: Division of Nursing, U.S. Bureau of Health Professions, Health Resources and Services Administration, U.S. Department of Health and Human Services, 1994.

Moses, E. B. *The Registered Nurse Population: Findings from the National Sample Survey of Registered Nurses, March 1996.* Rockville, Md.: Division of Nursing, U.S. Bureau of Health Professions, Health Resources and Services Administration, U.S. Department of Health and Human Services, 1997.

Munroe, D. J. "The Influence of Registered Nursing Staffing on the Quality of Nursing Home Care." *Research in Nursing and Health,* 1990, *13*(4), 263–270.

Murtaugh, C. M., Kemper, P., and Spillman, B. C. "The Risk of Nursing Home Use in Later Life." *Medical Care,* 1990, *28*(10), 952–962.

National Citizens Coalition for Nursing Home Reform. "Advocates Urge IOM Panel to Back Nurse Staffing Standards." *Quality Care Advocate,* Nov.-Dec. 1994.

Neu, C. R., and Harrison, S. C. *Posthospital Care Before and After the Medicare Prospective Payment System.* Health Care Financing Administration, USDHHS. Santa Monica, Calif.: Rand Corporation, 1988.

Nyman, J. A. "The Effect of Competition on Nursing Home Expenditures Under Prospective Reimbursement." *Health Services Research,* 1988a, *23,* 555.

Nyman, J. A. "Improving the Quality of Nursing Home Outcomes: Are Adequacy- or Incentive-Oriented Policies More Effective." *Medical Care,* 1988b, *26*(1), 158.

Nyman, J. A., Breaker, D. L., and Link, D. "Technical Efficiency in Nursing Home." *Medical Care,* 1990, *28*(6), 541–551.

Omnibus Budget Reconciliation Act of 1987. *Public Law 100–203. Subtitle C: Nursing Home Reform.* Signed by President, Washington, D.C., Dec. 22, 1987.

Ouslander, J., and Kane, R. "The Costs of Urinary Incontinence in Nursing Homes." *Medical Care,* 1984, *22,* 69–79.

Phillips, C. D., Hawes, C., and Fries, B. E. "Reducing the Use of Physical Restraints in Nursing Homes: Will It Increase Costs?" *American Journal of Public Health,* 1993, *83*(3), 342–348.

Ribeiro, B., and Smith, S. "Evaluation of Urinary Catheterization and Urinary Incontinence in a General Nursing Home Population." *Journal of the American Geriatrics Society,* 1985, *33,* 479–481.

Schneider, D. P., and others. "Case Mix for Nursing Home Payment: Resource Utilization Groups, Version II." *Health Care Financing Review,* 1988 Annual Supplement, pp. 39–52.

Shaughnessy, P. W., and Kramer, A. M. "Tradeoffs in Evaluating the Effectiveness of Nursing Home Care." In M. D. Mezey, J. E. Lynaugh, and M. M. Cartier (eds.), *Nursing Homes and Care: Lessons from Teaching Nursing Homes.* New York: Springer, 1989.

Shaughnessy, P. W., Schlenker, R. E., and Kramer, A. M. "Quality of Long-Term Care in Nursing Homes and Swing-Bed Hospitals." *Health Services Research,* 1990, *25*(1), 65–96.

Short, P. F., Kemper, P., Cornelius, L. J., and Walden, D. C. "Public and Private Responsibility for Financing Nursing-Home Care: The Effect of Medicaid Asset Spend-Down." *Milbank Quarterly,* 1992, *70*(2), 277–298.

Snow, K. I. *How States Determine Nursing Facility Eligibility for the Elderly: A National Survey.* Washington, D.C.: American Association of Retired Persons, 1995.

Spector, W. D., and Takada, H. A. "Characteristics of Nursing Homes That Affect Resident Outcomes." *Journal of Aging and Health,* 1991, *3*(4), 427–454.

Swan, J. H., DeWit, S., and Harrington, C. "State Medicaid Reimbursement Methods and Rates for Nursing Homes, 1993." Paper prepared for the Department of Housing and Urban Development and the Health Care Financing Administration. Wichita, Kans.: Wichita State University, 1995.

Swan, J. H., Harrington, C., and Grant, L. A. "State Medicaid Reimbursement for Nursing Homes, 1978–88." *Health Care Financing Review,* 1993, *14*(4), 111–131.

Turner, T. "Executive Committee of the Council on Nursing Administration." *Letter on Nursing Staffing.* Washington, D.C.: American Nurses Association, 1987.

U.S. Bureau of the Census. *Population Projections of the United States, by Age, Sex, Race, and Hispanic Origin: 1993 to 2050. Current Population Reports.* Prepared by J. C. Day. Pub. No. P25-1104. Washington, D.C.: U.S. Department of Commerce, 1993.

U.S. Department of Health and Human Services, Health Care Financing Administration. *Medicare and Medicaid Requirements for Long Term Care Facilities.* Final Rule. Federal Register, 1991.

U.S. General Accounting Office. "Report to the Chairman, Subcommittee on Health and Long-Term Care, Select Committee on Aging, House of Representatives." *Medicare and Medicaid: Stronger Enforcement of Nursing Home Requirements Needed.* Washington, D.C.: U.S. General Accounting Office, 1987.

U.S. House of Representatives, Committee on Ways and Means. *Overview of Entitlement Programs.* 1990 Green Book. Washington, D.C.: U.S. Government Printing Office, 1990, pp. 147–149.

U.S. Senate, Special Committee on Aging. *Nursing Home Care: The Unfinished Agenda.* (Special Hearing and Report, May 21, 1986). Washington, D.C.: U.S. Government Printing Office, 1986.

U.S. Senate Special Committee on Aging. *Reducing the Use of Chemical Restraints in Nursing Homes.* Workshop Before the Special Committee. SN 102–6. Washington, D.C.: U.S. Government Printing Office, 1991.

Weissert, W. G., and Musliner, M. C. *Access, Quality, and Cost Consequences of Case-Mix Adjusted Reimbursement for Nursing Homes.* No. 9109. Washington, D.C.: American Association of Retired Persons, 1992a.

Weissert, W. G., and Musliner, M. C. "Case Mix Adjusted Nursing-Home Reimbursement: A Critical Review of the Evidence." *Milbank Quarterly,* 1992b, *70*(3), 455–490.

Zedlewski, S. R., and McBride, T. D. "The Changing Profile of the Elderly: Effects on Future Long-Term Care Needs and Financing." *Milbank Quarterly,* 1992, *70*(2), 247–275.

Zimmerman, D. R. *Impact of New Regulations and Data Sources on Nursing Home Quality of Care.* Madison, Wis.: Center for Health Systems Research and Analysis, 1990.

Zimmerman, D. R., and others. "Development and Testing of Nursing Home Quality Indicators." *Health Care Financing Review,* 1995, *16*(4), 107–129.

Zinn, J. S. "Inter-SMSA Variation on Nursing Home Staffing and Management Practices." *Journal of Applied Gerontology,* 1993a, *12*(2), 206–224.

Zinn, J. S. "The Influence of Nurse Wage Differentials on Nursing Home Staffing and Resident Care Decisions." *The Gerontologist,* 1993b, *33*(6), 721–729.

Zinn, J. S., Aaronson, W. A., and Rosko, D. M. "The Use of Standardized Indicators as Quality Improvement Tools: An Application in Pennsylvania Nursing Homes." *American Journal of Medical Quality,* 1993a, *8,* 456–465.

Zinn, J. S., Aaronson, W. A., and Rosko, D. M. "Variations in Outcomes of Care Provided in Pennsylvania Nursing Homes: Facility and Environmental Correlates." *Medical Care,* 1993b, *31,* 475–487.

CHAPTER SEVEN

Changing Roles, Responsibilities, and Employment Patterns of Registered Nurses in Ambulatory Care Settings

Janis P. Bellack

In Chapter One, O'Neil identified the shift of care delivery from hospital to ambulatory settings as a major facet of the emerging health care environment. This shift has brought about an increase in the number of RNs working in free-standing ambulatory settings and in the number employed by hospitals in out-patient service units. The movement to ambulatory employment will be led by managed and integrated systems of care, which will deploy nurses in a variety of clinical services and managerial positions. Other areas of ambulatory employment will be schools, occupational health services, public clinics and services, and nursing centers. Ambulatory settings require nurses who are better prepared to exercise independent judgment and work in the community. These demands favor baccalaureate and advanced practice nursing professionals. Bellack enumerates the new skills and training RNs will need to meet the challenges of future practice in ambulatory settings.

Over the last decade, the growth and change in ambulatory care services has been nothing less than remarkable. Once confined to periodic health visits, minor episodic care, and follow-up treatment, ambulatory care services now encompass a broad range of medical, surgical, and behavioral care. The spectrum of services ranges from primary care delivered by individual providers to complex high-tech specialty services delivered by interdisciplinary teams of providers (Moreland, 1990). Today, ambulatory settings provide care to patients who tend to be sicker and who often require frequent and multiple visits.

Ambulatory care services are clearly the predominant growth sector in today's health care system. Regardless of how health care is financed in the future, there is little doubt that the trend toward managing health in settings other than acute care inpatient facilities will continue.

Ambulatory care encompasses direct health care services for individual patients and population groups that do not require overnight or longer stays. Services may be delivered in a variety of settings:

- Physician and managed care practices
- Outpatient diagnostic and surgery centers
- Nurse-managed or community nursing centers
- Publicly funded facilities such as county health departments, mental health centers, community health centers, rural health clinics, migrant health clinics, and Indian health clinics
- School and work settings
- Senior citizen and child day care centers
- Correctional facilities

These settings may range from being part of large, vertically integrated health care delivery systems to freestanding facilities.

FORCES INFLUENCING THE SHIFT TO AMBULATORY AND COMMUNITY-BASED CARE

With the advent of prospective payment for hospital services in the early 1980s, outpatient facilities increased in both number and scope, owing to shorter stays and earlier discharge of hospitalized patients, many of whom require intensive and frequent outpatient follow-up care. The shift from in-hospital to ambulatory health care services has been fueled further by the dramatic growth of managed care organizations described in Chapter One, which has increased competition among health care providers and accelerated pressure to deliver services in the least costly setting.

Perhaps the strongest driving force for expanding ambulatory care services has been the exorbitant increase in the daily cost of inpatient care, which rose 700 percent—from $667 to $4,572—between 1971 and 1989 (Droste, 1992). In 1982, per capita expenditures on in-hospital care in the United States were $570, up from $80 in 1966, the year following the initiation of Medicare. And between 1980 and 1989, Medicare enrollee payments doubled, increasing from $909 to $1,848 per enrollee, while supplementary medical insurance costs tripled.

The shift from inpatient to ambulatory care is transforming the health care system and creating new opportunities—and new demands—for nursing practice in settings other than the hospital. Although much of the nursing care delivered in ambulatory settings is similar to that provided in hospitals, the change in setting alters both the need for and scope of care.

SCOPE AND FUNDING OF AMBULATORY HEALTH CARE

The scope of health care delivered in ambulatory care settings runs the gamut from primary care to surgical intervention, and includes such services as the following:

- Health promotion and maintenance, health screening, and preventive care
- Diagnosis and treatment of acute episodic illness and injury
- Management of chronic illness
- Performance of invasive and noninvasive diagnostic and treatment procedures
- Surgery

These services are delivered in a variety of hospital-based and nonhospital-based ambulatory settings. Essentially, the ambulatory care setting is the linch-pin in an integrated delivery system, providing continuity of care management from home to outpatient settings, hospitals, and long-term care facilities, as needed.

The scope and availability of ambulatory services are tied directly to the revenue streams that underwrite their costs. Major sources of funding for ambulatory care include the following:

- Private insurers
- HMOs
- Federal government programs, including Medicare, Medicaid, categorical funding such as block grants and federally funded health centers and clinics, and graduate medical education support for teaching hospitals
- State and local dollars from city and county governments, school districts, and community-based nonprofit organizations
- Private foundations
- Industry and large businesses

A number of these funding sources have supported or mandated the use of nurses to provide selected ambulatory care services. Examples include Medicaid-funded early childhood screening programs, private foundation grants for nurse-managed school-based clinics, and rural health clinics. Some payers, however, prohibit patients from gaining direct access to advanced practice nurses for primary health care services, requiring instead that they be referred by a physician.

TRENDS IN AMBULATORY AND COMMUNITY-BASED CARE SERVICES

The extent of the shift from inpatient to outpatient care is evident in the available trend data. The American Hospital Association (AHA) reported that in 1970, the average daily inpatient census in all U.S. hospitals was nearly 1.3 million. By 1980, it had dropped to 1 million, and by 1990 to less than 850,000 (American Hospital Association, 1981, 1990; Droste, 1992), despite a concomitant 25 percent increase in the U.S. population. The total number of annual inpatient days declined from 273,200 in 1983 to 215,900 by 1993, a 21 percent drop (Wunderlich, Sloan, and Davis, 1996).

During these same periods, the number of annual outpatient visits in all U.S. hospitals increased 75 percent (American Hospital Association, 1981, 1990; Wunderlich, Sloan, and Davis, 1996). In one year alone (1994–95), outpatient clinic visits in community hospitals increased 16.5 percent (Wunderlich, Sloan, and Davis, 1996). Furthermore, outpatient revenues continue to climb as a proportion of total hospital-based revenues (Fraser, Lane, Linne, and Jones, 1993).

In 1980, half of all U.S. hospitals reported having organized outpatient services. By 1989, that number had increased to 70 percent. Even more dramatic was the increase in outpatient surgery services, which was not even included as a reporting category in the 1980 AHA survey. By 1990, 84 percent of all hospitals reported providing outpatient surgery services. The American College of Surgeons (1988) reported that the annual number of surgical procedures performed in hospital outpatient settings rose from 3.2 million in 1980 to 8.7 million in 1986, and represented over 40 percent of all surgical procedures performed by hospitals in 1986. By 1991, over half of all surgeries were being performed on an outpatient basis, and the total number had increased to nearly 12 million annually (Fraser, Lane, Linne, and Jones, 1993). Furthermore, both the number of freestanding ambulatory surgery centers and the number of procedures they performed (see Figure 7.1) quadrupled between 1985 and 1993 (SMG Marketing Group, 1994).

The AHA surveys also reveal that by 1989, new reporting categories had been added for "women's center/health services," "reproductive health services," and "health promotion services," further evidence of the expanding scope of ambulatory care (American Hospital Association, 1981, 1990). These services, respectively, were offered by 17.4 percent, 34.7 percent, and 83.6 percent of all U.S. hospitals. Between 1986 and 1990, the number of U.S. community hospitals offering "patient education services" increased by one-third, and those offering "community health promotion programs" increased 40 percent. By 1990, nearly eight out of ten community hospitals were offering community health promotion programs (Fraser, Lane, Linne, and Jones, 1993).

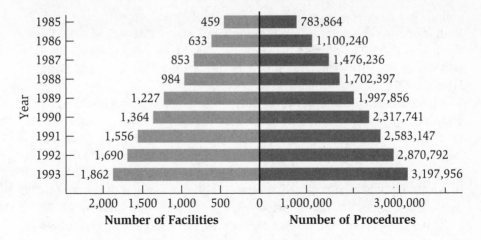

Figure 7.1. Growth of Freestanding Ambulatory Surgical Centers.

Source: SMG Marketing Group, 1994

The increasing emphasis that hospitals are placing on health promotion and risk reduction reflects a trend toward greater involvement in providing outreach, education, and support services for the community. Typical services include weight management, physical fitness, smoking cessation, alcohol and drug abuse education, injury prevention, family planning, prenatal and parenting education, child and spouse abuse prevention, stress management, and education for specific health problems. The delivery of such services promotes a positive image for community hospitals and helps them attract patients in a competitive health care market. As managed care networks and integrated delivery systems form, health promotion services—offered primarily in ambulatory and community-based health care settings—will likely become increasingly vital components of the services offered by these systems. These health promotion efforts are consistent with the value improvement stage of managed care described in Chapter Four, in which heightened attention to the health promotion needs of individuals fosters awareness of the social determinants of health, prompting movement toward the third (health improvement) stage of managed care.

NURSING EMPLOYMENT AND PRACTICE
IN AMBULATORY CARE: DRIVING FORCES AND BARRIERS

Not surprisingly, nursing employment patterns have changed with the shift of health care to ambulatory settings, both in numbers of RNs employed and the settings that employ them. The same forces that are driving the expansion of ambulatory care services are creating new employment opportunities for RNs. With increasing acceptance—by consumers and payers alike—of advanced practice nurses (APNs) as primary care providers, managed care organizations have begun to employ APNs in large numbers (Bednash, 1996; Green and Conway-Welch, 1995).

As Fralic notes in Chapter Five, during the 1980s the number of full-time equivalent RNs employed by hospitals increased significantly despite the closure and downsizing of a large number of hospitals. This paradox resulted largely from the increased acuity of hospitalized patients and the move to primary nursing and all-RN staffing. However, some of the increase in hospital-based RN employment is clearly the result of the expansion of hospital-based outpatient services, including invasive diagnostic procedures and surgery.

By the early 1990s, ambulatory settings employed large numbers of RNs. As noted in Chapter Two, hospital-based outpatient departments experienced a 100 percent increase in RN employment between 1988 and 1996 (Moses, 1997), accompanied by an additional 15 percent increase in RNs employed in non-hospital ambulatory care settings (Wunderlich, Sloan, and Davis, 1996). In addition, the number of newly licensed RN graduates employed in community-based settings increased 5 percent and 11 percent, respectively, over the previous two years (American Nurses Association, 1995).

According to the National Sample Survey of RNs, 21.6 percent of the total RN workforce was employed in ambulatory or community-public health care settings by 1996 (Moses, 1997). However, this percentage is probably substantially higher than reported, because the survey did not obtain information about the specific settings in which hospital-based nurses were practicing. Given the significant increase in employment of RNs in hospital-based outpatient departments reported by Wunderlich, Sloan, and Davis (1996), many RNs employed by hospitals clearly are working in ambulatory care.

Haas and Hackbarth (1995a) point out, "Since the value of prevention has finally been noticed by mainstream policymakers, the opportunities for ambulatory staff nurses in this area should be limitless" (p. 238). The question remains, however, whether substantial numbers of employers, such as HMOs, physician group practices, and state and federal guarantors of health care for the poor and uninsured will recognize the value and cost-effectiveness of employing RNs and APNs to provide a selected range of ambulatory care services.

Several barriers to expanded employment and utilization of nurses in ambulatory care settings continue to exist:

- State practice acts that restrict the scope and autonomy of nurses, especially APNs
- The current monopoly by physicians on care coordination and reimbursement

- An oversupply of physicians
- Restrictive insurance and reimbursement regulations
- The "bottom line" mentality of most managed care organizations, including the desire to employ the least expensive provider to fulfill roles and functions traditionally associated with nursing
- The current medical model organization of most ambulatory care settings, which undervalues nursing's holistic approach to care
- Poor role differentiation within nursing
- Inadequate educational preparation for new nursing roles in ambulatory care
- Administrative and organizational obstacles, such as limited work space, limited access to communication and information management equipment (telephones, computers, and so forth), lack of time for patient teaching and follow-up, inadequate staff support, and excessive paperwork

Despite these barriers, it is likely that nurses will be utilized increasingly for ambulatory care roles. Weiner (1995) notes that the current demand for "mid-level practitioners"—nurse midwives, nurse practitioners, and physician assistants—in HMOs exceeds the current supply. Numerous studies confirm consumer satisfaction with the care provided by APNs (Office of Technology Assessment, 1986), and payers prefer their lower costs compared with family physicians who provide essentially the same scope of services. In fact, Beckham (1996) points out that primary care physicians are "expensive middlemen," and says there is compelling evidence that health plans will move from a "gate-keeper" model controlled by primary care physicians to a "gateway" model, in which APNs and physician assistants provide primary care services and refer patients directly to specialist care.

However, the ideal size, skill mix, and roles of the ambulatory care nursing workforce have yet to be determined. Although the desired nurse staffing mix in acute care settings, depending on patient acuity, has been estimated at 70–80 percent RNs, with the balance in unlicensed assistive personnel (Sovie, 1995), no similar estimate has yet been projected for ambulatory care settings.

OPPORTUNITIES FOR EXPANDED NURSE EMPLOYMENT IN AMBULATORY CARE

Because of the dramatic shift to managed care and integrated delivery systems, these systems—which include many physician office practices—are likely to provide the greatest potential in the future for nurse employment in ambulatory care. Other opportunities include occupational and school health services, publicly funded ambulatory care sites, and such alternative ambulatory services as community nursing centers.

Managed Care and Integrated Delivery Systems

As O'Neil notes in Chapter One, managed care has emerged over the last decade as the dominant means for controlling costs while maintaining the quality of health care services. In principle, managed care—with its emphasis on prevention, early intervention, and continuity of care—has the potential to increase employment opportunities in ambulatory care settings for both RNs and APNs. Care provided by a cadre of nurses can help control costs, reduce the need for hospitalization (or rehospitalization), and improve health outcomes for a managed care population (American Nurses Association, 1995). Although in 1996 only 1 percent of the RN population was employed in HMOs (Moses, 1997), demand for RNs in managed care organizations will increase as those organizations expand their home health, patient education, self-care programs, and prevention and early detection services. This especially will hold true when managed care systems "mature to the point where [they] compete not only on cost, but on quality of care as well" (American Nurses Association, 1995, p. 5).

Health plans also are employing RNs to respond to consumer inquiries on the telephone, apply clinical pathways over the phone, and when needed, direct patients to a specialist. Beckham (1996) notes this trend is "particularly good news for nurses, who are likely to continue to find their ranks thinned in acute-care settings. For many nurses, [this] will provide an opportunity to deliver care with the authority and responsiveness they've long sought but could never achieve in the . . . hierarchies of the hospital" (p. 63).

Physician Office Practices

Growth in managed care can be expected to have a direct impact on RN employment in physician office practices as well. In 1996, 5.4 percent (114,258) of the RN workforce was employed in physician office practices, which included solo, partnership, and group practices, freestanding clinics, and nonhospital-based ambulatory surgical and diagnostic centers (Moses, 1997). An additional 19,003 RNs were employed in mixed professional practice groups. The Bureau of Labor Statistics predicts a 24 percent increase between 1994 and 2005 in the number of RNs working in physician offices, given the increasing size and aging of the U.S. population and the expected continuing shift to managed care.

However, the potential for expanded RN employment in physician office practices remains uncertain, because managed care has a direct impact on the traditional model of the physician as employer. Decisions about nurse staffing in physician offices are no longer made exclusively by the physicians practicing in them. As more practices are purchased by or choose to affiliate with integrated delivery systems or participate in managed risk contracts, opportunities for APNs and RNs to provide primary care services and nurse-managed specialty services in ambulatory care group practices are likely to increase. Physician receptivity and the desire of managed care networks to employ the least expensive, qualified health care worker will be key variables that can influence—both favorably and unfavorably—employment opportunities for RNs in these settings.

School Health Services

There is tremendous potential for schools to become the primary site of routine health care for a majority of the nation's children. Most of this care could be provided by RNs and APNs. School settings are a natural place to deliver health care because 95 percent of the nation's children between five and eighteen years of age attend school.

School-based health services keep children healthy and in school, thus reducing health care costs and improving educational outcomes (Passarelli, 1994; Yates, 1994). Yates (1994) notes that school-based health services "meet and promote the health needs of students . . . and families by eliminating obstacles of lack of transportation, inconvenient scheduling, economic constraints, and unacceptability of services in traditional health care systems" (p. 12). School health services typically focus on promoting health, preventing disease and injury, helping children become active and knowledgeable partners in their health care, and reducing fragmentation of care for the school-age population. Services may include periodic or sports physical exams, routine laboratory tests, treatment of minor illness and injury, administration of medications, health education, health screening, counseling, and referral, all of which can be provided in school settings.

School-based health services also can provide needed care for children with chronic illness or disability. With the passage of federal legislation in 1975 (P. L. 94–142, Handicapped Children Act) mandating education in "the least restrictive environment," and the more recent Americans with Disabilities Act (P. L. 101–336), increasing numbers of children with chronic illness and disability are attending mainstream schools. Such children often require special health services during school hours, and school-based nurses can provide needed care, prevent expensive complications, and help educate teachers and staff about an ill or disabled child's special needs.

School-based nurses or school-based/school-linked health centers or clinics (SB/SLHCs) provide a comprehensive array of health services, and as such are capable of addressing the major primary health care needs of the school populations they serve. In 1992, the Center for Population Options reported 510 SB/SLHCs in forty-one states, Guam, and Puerto Rico; 415 were school-based (located in the school or on school grounds), and 95 were school-linked clinics (located off school grounds but usually within walking distance).

Currently, however, school-based health services are reaching less than 1 percent of the school-age population (Waszak and Neidell, 1991). Furthermore, school health services tend to be offered in schools with high minority enrollments, often the most underserved, underfunded, and hard to reach school-age populations. Provision of on-site health care services to children and adolescents to keep them healthy, help them develop lifelong positive health habits, treat minor illness and injury, and manage chronic illness and disability in the community—rather than in more costly hospital-based or other ambulatory clinic settings—can help control health care costs, now and in the future, for this population.

A number of barriers—political, economic, and regulatory—prevent nurses from providing health services for larger numbers of school-age children. The greatest proportion of fiscal support for school health services is provided by state health and human service departments, but most also receive funds from federal block grants, local monies, and private foundations. Private foundation funding of SBHCs declined substantially in the late 1980s, from 41 percent of the average SBHC's budget in 1987 to 19 percent in 1989 (Waszak and Neidell, 1991). Continuation funding has been particularly scarce, with few school-based clinics receiving other than in-kind support from local budgets. Unfortunately, school districts with the greatest need for health services also are those with the lowest tax base and per-pupil funding.

Only a small fraction of RNs are employed in school-based settings: 2.5 percent (53,709) in 1996 (Moses, 1997). The vast majority (89 percent) worked in public schools, providing health services for an entire school or, in many instances, for students in more than one school. An additional 9,222 RNs (less than 1 percent of the workforce) were employed by colleges or universities to provide student health services.

Until payers—both public and private—are willing to fund preventive and early treatment services in schools, it is unlikely that school health services will expand in any significant way or provide increased opportunities for RN employment in the near future. Furthermore, school nurse salaries are among the lowest in the profession, making it difficult to attract RNs accustomed to the higher pay scales available in other settings.

Occupational Health Services

Work settings are more likely to provide on-site health care services and do not face the same political and economic obstacles that schools do. In fact, there are strong economic incentives for offering on-site health services in the work setting. Corporations and businesses currently pay for health care for 150 million Americans, spending more than $3,000 per employee in 1990 (Burgel, 1993). From 1981 to 1983, 3.8 percent of businesses with fewer than 100 employees provided on-site health services, while 32 percent of those with 100 to 499 employees did so, as did 87 percent of those with 500 or more employees (U.S. Department of Health and Human Services, 1988). Employers increasingly are offering such services, with 90 percent of Fortune 500 companies reporting they employ registered nurses (Lusk, Disch, and Barkauskas, 1988).

Numerous studies have demonstrated the health and cost benefits of providing on-site occupational health nursing services (Bey, McGovern, and Foley, 1988; Burgel, 1993; Lusk, Disch, and Barkauskas, 1988; Touger and Butts, 1989; U.S. Department of Health and Human Services, National Institute of Occupational Health and Safety, 1980). Given the economic and health benefits that derive from on-site services, and the fact that occupational health nurses—especially those prepared at the advanced practice level—can provide the full scope of services needed, the potential for continued expansion of this ambulatory nursing role is great. Further, companies may be propelled in the future to extend their worksite health services to the dependents of their employees—at the worksite, in schools and day care centers, or in satellite clinics, realizing further health and cost benefits for employers as well as employees and their families.

Occupational health settings employed an estimated 21,575 (1 percent) of RNs in 1996, the majority of whom work in private industry (Burgel, 1993; Moses, 1997). Occupational health nurses provide wellness care, prevent work-related illness and injury, implement employee assistance programs, conduct health risk appraisals and screening, conduct surveillance to prevent and detect hazardous exposure, and provide case management services. Nurses are the sole health care providers in 60 percent of companies that employ occupational health nurses (Burgel, 1993).

Publicly Funded Ambulatory Care Services

A variety of publicly funded settings provide ambulatory health care services, generally for rural, underserved, poor, and uninsured populations. These include federally designated community health centers, rural health clinics, migrant health clinics, and Indian health clinics, and state, city, or county public health departments. They also include local, state, and federal correctional facilities. Such settings often employ advanced practice nurses, as well as RNs, LPNs and LVNs, and unlicensed assistive personnel (UAPs).

Nearly 6 percent of the RN workforce is employed in publicly funded ambulatory care settings. Approximately 100,000 of them practice in such settings as health departments, neighborhood health centers, family planning centers, day care centers, retirement community centers, community mental health services, and outpatient substance abuse facilities (Moses, 1997). An additional 11,911 RNs provide health care services to inmates in city and county jails and state and federal prisons.

The shift to early hospital discharge and outpatient follow-up has added new demands for ambulatory health care services, especially for high-risk and uninsured populations (Hockey, 1995). Additional resources—both human and fiscal—will be needed to ensure that adequate services are available in ambulatory care settings to prevent complications, rehospitalization, and the use of high-cost emergency room services. RNs and APNs can provide the health care services needed by these groups and maintain quality of care while reducing costs. However, nursing positions in ambulatory sites that care for high-risk populations are unlikely to expand in the foreseeable future; in fact, indications are they may be reduced due to cuts in federal and state programs.

Nursing Centers

Nursing centers—also called nurse-managed centers or community nursing centers—have emerged over the last two decades as alternative ambulatory health care delivery settings (Barger, 1995). Many nursing centers are affiliated with schools of nursing and serve as practice sites for faculty and clinical learning sites for students.

By 1992, there were 250 documented ambulatory care facilities that met the established criteria for a nursing center (Knauth, 1994). Nursing centers are characterized by the following (Barger, 1995; Knauth, 1994; National League for Nursing, 1992):

- Direct client access to nursing services
- A nurse in the chief executive position who retains overall accountability for the center
- A nursing staff that is accountable and responsible for patient care and professional practice
- Client-centered patient care services that are reimbursed at a reasonable fee
- A nursing model of care that emphasizes diagnostic and treatment services that promote health and optimal functioning

Depending on the client population served and state regulations, a number of nursing centers also employ other health professionals, including physicians or such allied health professionals as social workers and nutritionists, to provide back-up coverage, supplemental services, and consultation. Nursing centers may be freestanding, affiliated with a university nursing school, or linked with other health agencies such as home health, long-term care settings, or hospitals.

Services provided by nursing centers include physical, developmental, and health risk appraisal, health education and risk reduction, diagnosis and treatment of acute episodic illness, management of chronic illness, psychosocial counseling, case management, and referral (Barger, 1995; Phillips and Steel,

1994). Although nursing centers may be viewed as competition by other providers, especially physicians, Phillips and Steel believe that nursing centers are "a new, complimentary [sic], community-based alternative" (1994, p. 89) with a distinct scope of services that is client-centered and rooted in nursing's commitment to provide care for the community, especially populations that otherwise would not have access to health services (Barger, 1995). A number of nursing centers target specific patient populations. These include pregnant women, children, persons living in low-income housing projects, the elderly, persons with AIDS, persons in need of cardiac rehabilitation, the homeless, university students and faculty, and prison inmates (Barger, 1995; Phillips and Steel, 1994).

Most nursing centers employ both RNs and APNs, including nurse practitioners, certified nurse midwives, and clinical nurse specialists (Phillips and Steel, 1994). However, the number of nurses who currently practice in these and other nurse-based practice settings, including solo and group practices, is very small (less than one-half of 1 percent) (Moses, 1997). Although nursing centers are supported by a variety of funding sources, including federal and foundation grants, universities, contributions, and direct reimbursement, many have an unstable funding base, and a number have been forced to close because of insufficient or discontinued funding (Barger, 1995).

There is some evidence of interest in developing nursing centers as HMOs (Lamb, 1994). Etheridge (1991) describes the success of a nursing HMO that provided services to Medicare recipients under a capitated plan. This is the first such model for direct contracting with payers to provide an agreed-upon set of integrated, community-based nursing services. Services include case management, home health, and respite care.

In the early 1990s, the Health Care Financing Administration (HCFA) funded four demonstration sites of community nursing organizations (CNOs) to provide capitated nurse-managed ambulatory and community-based health services for groups of Medicare beneficiaries (Lamb, 1994). These CNOs provided home health, case management, therapy services, emergency transport, prosthetic devices, and medical equipment. Lamb notes, "The cornerstones of the CNO system are direct access to professional nursing care, neighborhood and home-based service delivery, emphasis on health promotion and prevention services, and flexible authorization of covered services based on client need" (p. 9).

In the managed care marketplace, nursing centers have the potential to "become the backbone of a coordinated, community-based health system that will focus on prevention and early treatment of common problems" (Jenkins and Torrisi, 1995, p. 123). Centers that employ APNs can provide comprehensive, high-quality, cost-effective primary health care services to their client populations. As with the CNO demonstration sites, nursing centers may be able to ensure their future viability by contracting directly with state and private managed care plans, thus reducing health care costs to payers and beneficiaries (Green and Conway-Welch, 1995; Jenkins and Torrisi, 1995; Torrisi, 1994).

Phillips and Steel (1994) suggest removing legal barriers to practice and direct reimbursement for nursing services to ensure the continuance and expansion of nursing centers in the future. In the foreseeable future, however, it is unlikely that nursing centers will provide significant employment opportunities for hospital-displaced nurses because they currently provide a very small volume of services.

NURSING ROLES IN AMBULATORY CARE

The shift of health care to ambulatory settings is creating new opportunities for nurses. The care delivered in these settings, and therefore the roles and functions of the nurses who work in them, are influenced by the unique characteristics of the ambulatory settings themselves. Among these are the following (Curran, 1995):

- Rapid work pace and client turnover
- Brevity of patient encounters (minutes to hours instead of days and weeks)
- Importance of triage, including telephone triage
- Need for effective coordination with other care delivery settings (seamless care)
- Different workforce skill mix (typically fewer RNs)
- Greater delegation and supervision of nonprofessional staff
- Greater autonomy in decision making
- Fewer immediate resources—such as house staff or even supplies—for managing care.

Historically, RNs have been underutilized in ambulatory care settings. A study of a broad, representative sample of nurses employed in ambulatory care settings in university hospitals, community hospitals, physician group practices, and HMOs revealed that the least frequently performed activities were in the most complex categories: care coordination and expert practice (Hackbarth, Haas, Kavanagh, and Vlasses, 1995). Instead, staff nurses in the study reported "more frequent performance of lower-level dimensions and less frequent performance of dimensions requiring disciplinary knowledge and critical thinking, despite the growing complexity of care in ambulatory settings" (p. 94). These findings lend credence to the notion that, at the present time, RNs in ambulatory care settings are not being utilized appropriately, cost-effectively, or to their full capabilities.

Building on Verran's (1981) earlier research on the dimensions of the staff nurse role in ambulatory care, Hackbarth, Haas, Kavanagh, and Vlasses (1995) delineated eight core dimensions of the current clinical practice role, depicted in Table 7.1. Haas and Hackbarth (1995a) subsequently reported that the ambulatory care nurses in their sample projected several significant role changes in the future. Specifically, study participants predicted an expansion of their client teaching role to include assessment of learning needs and follow-up of client outcomes. The expert practice role is projected to encompass community outreach activities, including provision of primary care services, group education in the community, and home follow-up. Also, an entirely new role category was projected—high-tech procedures—which includes such advanced technical skills as administration of blood and blood products, performance of complex treatments, and monitoring clients before and after invasive diagnostic or surgical procedures.

Haas and Hackbarth's (1995a) sample also defined the "ideal role" for ambulatory care nurses to include professional autonomy, use of nursing knowledge, direct caregiving, client and family teaching, collaboration and colleagueship with physicians and other providers, community outreach, primary prevention, case management, and fewer nonprofessional duties such as clerical work. These authors conclude that "nurses . . . want to actively apply the full scope of professional nursing knowledge and clinical skills in ambulatory settings in the future. The concept of nurses practicing with increased autonomy, emphasizing health promotion and health teaching as well as hands-on care in primary health care settings, is also consistent with many recommendations for health care reorganization" (p. 235).

In the future, RNs who practice in ambulatory care are likely to be less engaged in direct care provision, unless they are practicing in advanced practice roles. Instead, RNs are assuming expanded responsibilities for management and coordination of personnel, services, data, and resources as well as patient and family education, while technical and support roles in the ambulatory setting are likely to be filled by LPNs and UAPs (American Nurses Association, 1995; Loveridge, 1995; H. Evert and J. Peacock-Moye, personal communication, March 26, 1996; M. Bradley, personal communication, April 18, 1996). RNs are becoming increasingly responsible for coordinating care for groups of patients across delivery settings, from ambulatory care to home health to hospital care. In this new management role, ambulatory care RNs will be held accountable—as members of the professional team—for service delivery and clinical outcomes.

Case management is another role that RNs may be increasingly called upon to perform. Examples include managing care in such areas as diabetes education, pain management, cardiac rehabilitation, infusion therapy, and communicable

Table 7.1. Core Dimensions of the RN Clinical Practice Role in Ambulatory Care.

*Enabling operations—measure vital signs, maintain traffic flow, transport clients, maintain space/equipment and a safe work environment, order supplies, obtain records.

*Technical procedures—prepare client, chaperone and assist with procedures, witness informed consent, collect specimens, administer oral/IM medications.

*Nursing process—obtain patient history, assess learning needs, develop care plan, evaluate client care outcomes, document care.

*Telephone communications—triage, call pharmacy with prescriptions, call client with test results, home care follow-up.

*Advocacy—promote positive public relations, act as client advocate, inform client of rights, triage client to appropriate provider.

*Teaching—instruct on treatment, instruct on home- or self-care.

*High-tech procedures—administer IV therapy and blood/blood products, perform complex treatments, monitor clients before and after procedures.

*Care coordination—coordinate care, initiate referrals, identify community resources, provide long-term supportive relationship.

*Expert practice/community outreach—possess expertise in advanced nursing practice, precept students, provide inservice education, serve as advanced nurse resource, independently provide primary care, organize and conduct group teaching, participate in community outreach, follow up clients in the home.

Sources: Hackbarth, D. P., Haas, S. A., Kavanagh, J. A., and Vlasses, F. *Nursing Economic$,* 1995, *13*(2), p. 92 and Haas, S. A., and Hackbarth, D. P. *Nursing Economic$,* 1995, *13*(4), p. 233. Reprinted with permission of the publisher, Janetti Publications, Inc., East Holly Avenue, Box 56, Pitman, NJ 08071–0056 (Phone: 609–256–2300).

diseases. RNs will be needed to develop and oversee critical pathways for these client groups to achieve desired outcomes, control costs, improve provider efficiency, and enhance patient satisfaction. RN case managers will be especially critical in managing care for low-income populations, who may have low literacy skills and who may need assistance negotiating the health care system and accessing community resources. RNs must be able to coordinate and interface effectively with home care and other community-based services, as well as consult with inpatient units when patients are hospitalized.

There is some evidence that RNs, especially those with baccalaureate and advanced degrees, will be employed in greater numbers to work with high-risk outpatient populations and in ambulatory settings that are highly intense and complex, such as ambulatory surgery and outpatient diagnostic centers (L. Bonadonna, personal communication, April 1996; H. Evert and J. Peacock-Moye, personal communication, March 1996; K. Weaver, personal communication, April 1996). Patients in the ambulatory diagnostic or surgery setting frequently have high acuity levels, and increasingly complex procedures are being performed on an outpatient basis, necessitating a higher ratio of RNs to other nursing personnel.

In the outpatient diagnostic or surgery setting, RNs are expected to perform a range of services that require astute assessment and clinical judgment skills, application of clinical practice guidelines and professional care standards, patient and family education and support, effective communication, collaboration and team skills, use of critical pathways and continuous improvement, and flexibility and adaptability in environments of rapid change. LPNs and UAPs generally lack the knowledge and clinical judgment skills to perform these roles, although they can be effective care partners with RNs in carrying out delegated tasks (Haas and Hackbarth, 1995a). APNs also are being utilized as cost-effective providers in these high-intensity ambulatory settings, conducting preoperative physical exams, monitoring patient recovery, prescribing pain medications, and writing discharge and follow-up treatment orders.

Many ambulatory care functions can be performed safely by LPNs or LVNs and UAPs, using established protocols, including certain delegated technical procedures, telephone triage, medication administration, and some patient education. In high-volume, low-intensity primary care settings with physicians or APNs on site, administrators see little need for the RN role (M. Bradley, personal communication, April 18, 1996; H. Evert and J. Peacock-Moye, personal communication, March 26, 1996). Reliable data are not yet available to know what effect the provision of nursing and patient support services by LPNs and UAPs in low-intensity primary care settings has on patient outcomes and cost. Also, the extent to which LPNs and UAPs are utilized in ambulatory care will vary from state to state, depending on licensure and regulatory statutes, and from organization to organization, depending on mission, values, and target population.

Practice Roles in Ambulatory Care

Traditionally, ambulatory care services have been organized in a medical model in which physicians provide reimbursable care to individuals who need diagnostic and treatment services for a variety of diseases (Haas, Hackbarth, Kavanagh, and Vlasses, 1995). Nurses, on the other hand, are educated to care for the whole person in the context of family and community. They are prepared specifically to promote health and prevent illness, assess health status and risks, provide health education to individuals and groups, and help patients manage and cope with actual or potential health problems, in a variety of settings (American Nurses Association, 1995; Haas, Hackbarth, Kavanagh, and Vlasses, 1995). These skills are particularly suited to the increasing emphasis placed on health promotion, health education, and out-of-hospital treatment and management of illness in a managed care environment. In fact, ambulatory care, with its focus on providing a full scope of health care services, provides numerous opportunities for nurses to use their patient education and supportive care skills in ways that are congruent with their educational preparation.

There are tremendous opportunities for RNs to be utilized more appropriately and effectively in ambulatory settings, with the potential for greater professional satisfaction and high-quality care at affordable prices. Currently, RNs in ambulatory care are spending time in activities that could be delegated safely and appropriately to LPNs or LVNs and UAPs. Many of the enabling operations and technical procedures (see Table 7.1) could be performed by others under RN supervision, freeing RNs to concentrate on the more complex role dimensions that require clinical judgment, collaboration, communication, and other higher-level professional skills. Innovative ambulatory care providers are already implementing these changes, but it remains to be seen whether the majority will follow.

Advanced Nursing Practice in Ambulatory Care

Advanced practice nurses may have the greatest potential for expanded employment in ambulatory care. The majority are prepared to work in primary and ambulatory care settings as generalists or specialists. Moreover, there is widespread recognition and acceptance of the ability of APNs to provide 60 to 80 percent of essential primary care services (Bednash, 1996; Office of Technology Assessment, 1986). Further, APNs do so in safe, effective ways and at lower cost than primary care physicians (Beckham, 1996; Bednash, 1996). Bednash concludes, "As the care delivery system continues its dramatic movement to a structure organized around principles of cost and appropriateness, the need for these clinicians will grow, helping put the highest quality, lowest cost provider next to the patient" (1996, p. 216). However, Bednash cautions that APNs are not simply less expensive substitutes for primary care physicians. Though APNs have been shown to have clinical knowledge comparable to primary care physicians, they also are more effective in addressing health promotion and improving patients' functional status, with greater patient satisfaction and compliance with care (Office of Technology Assessment, 1986).

HMOs already employ or contract with practices that include significant numbers of APNs (Haas and Hackbarth, 1995a). Some HMO contracts now allow enrollees to select APNs as their primary care providers. Whether other ambulatory care settings or managed care plans will follow suit remains to be seen. APNs are more likely to be employed in settings that provide care for rural and underserved populations. In fact, the majority of APNs who currently practice in primary health care settings are employed by community health centers, rural health clinics, migrant health centers, nursing centers, and HMOs (American Nurses Association, 1995; Haas and Hackbarth, 1995a).

As with RNs, APNs often are underutilized, given their preparation and capabilities. Frampton and Wall (1994) found that APNs were managing only 25 percent of all patient visits in HMO practices, whereas they had the ability to manage 60 percent. Perhaps the most desirable and cost-effective model is a collaborative practice model in which primary care physicians and APNs practice as a team to provide comprehensive care for a defined population or panel of patients.

Since 1993, when federal health care reform failed and state and private efforts to control health care costs began to escalate, demand for APNs appears to be growing. Numerous reports have called for training increased numbers of advanced practice nurses to meet the public's needs for primary health care and for removing regulatory barriers so they can practice to their full capability (American Academy of Nursing, 1993; Finocchio and others, 1995; National League for Nursing, 1991, 1993; O'Neil, 1993; Pew Health Professions Commission Advisory Panel, 1995).

Role Differentiation in Ambulatory Care

A major issue that remains to be addressed is the need for clear role differentiation. What are the appropriate roles and responsibilities in the ambulatory care setting for physicians, APNs, RNs, LPNs and LVNs, and UAPs? Issues of educational preparation, disciplinary focus (that is, medical model versus holistic model), experience, and cost must be considered. The goal should be employment of the most appropriate provider to ensure quality outcomes for the lowest cost.

In specialty clinics, high-tech diagnostic centers, and outpatient surgery centers, specialty physicians will, of course, be the core providers. By contrast, in primary care and some acute care settings, APNs can provide the same range of medical services as physicians while adding the holistic nursing dimension to patient care. Highly paid physicians should care for the 20–30 percent of primary care patients whose health care needs cannot be addressed fully by an APN. Neither physicians nor APNs, however, should be spending valuable time engaged in activities that can just as effectively be carried out by an appropriately prepared RN—for example, case management, community outreach, group teaching, delegation of care, and supervision of LPNs and LVNs and unlicensed personnel.

In the same vein, RNs should be used in appropriate and cost-effective ways, taking into account their educational preparation and experience. RNs prepared at the baccalaureate level can provide health promotion and screening, care coordination, case management, community outreach, group teaching, follow-up and referral, continuous improvement, and resource management. Although RNs who have an associate degree or diploma are not prepared to provide these more complex services, they can be utilized effectively to assess patients, manage patient flow, administer medications and treatments, document care, provide telephone counseling using established protocols, and instruct patients on home care. Duties that can be safely and effectively carried out by less skilled nursing personnel, such as LPNs, LVNs, and UAPs, should be delegated to them (Cohen, 1996). Such duties include the enabling operations and some of the technical procedures defined by Hackbarth, Haas, Kavanagh, and Vlasses (1995).

Haas and Hackbarth (1995b) call for the development of professional standards, clinical ladders, and quality improvement processes to support new models of nursing care delivery in ambulatory care. Such models would specify competencies and differentiate roles of nurses who practice in ambulatory care, with the potential for improved quality and cost-effectiveness of care. The unique characteristics of the ambulatory care setting requires nurses who work in these settings to possess certain essential competencies:

- Excellent communication and interpersonal skills, that is, "access, attitude, and affability," and customer responsiveness

- Effective and culturally competent patient-family education and support skills

- Ability to think critically and quickly—to set priorities, grasp the big picture, and make accurate clinical judgments

- Up-to-date clinical skills, including "focused and fast" assessment and triage skills

- Excellent organizational skills—to keep patient flow moving, minimize inefficiencies, and manage time and multiple priorities efficiently

- Knowledge of resources in the health care system and the community and of how to access them and use them wisely

- Effective use of information resources, including electronic information and communication technologies

- Ability to work cooperatively and collaboratively in teams
- Acceptance of accountability for quality of care delivered, patient satisfaction, patient outcomes, and cost-effective use of resources
- Superb flexibility, adaptability, and willingness to embrace change
- Commitment to lifelong learning

As managed care moves to a focus on managing *care* rather than *cost* and provides incentives for keeping people well or effectively managing their chronic diseases, there will be an increasing need for nurses with the broadened competencies consistent with those recommended by the Pew Health Professions Commission (1995):

- Providing integrated health services
- Working in interdisciplinary teams
- Emphasizing health promotion and disease prevention
- Functioning in managed care environments
- Evaluating quality and cost of health care

Such competencies typically are acquired in baccalaureate and higher degree programs.

Nurses prepared at the baccalaureate level are likely to be well suited for future practice roles in ambulatory care settings. A substantial portion of the curriculum in BSN programs focuses on primary prevention, health screening, patient and family education, community and population health, care coordination and management, and research utilization, all of which apply directly to ambulatory care. BSN graduates acquire a foundation that readies them to provide and manage a variety of ambulatory health care services, including worksite and school-based wellness programs, clinics to monitor groups of healthy clients or coordinate care for a specific population of chronically ill patients, immunization programs, telephone counseling and triage, patient and community education classes, and health screening and referral. Conversely, associate degree and diploma education programs primarily prepare graduates to provide direct care for individuals and groups in acute care settings. Although students in these programs may have some experiences in ambulatory care, the experiences tend to be limited to observation, and students are not usually expected to acquire the knowledge or skills necessary for practice in ambulatory settings.

Use of APNs for some ambulatory care roles is neither cost-effective nor ideally suited to their role preparation and advanced practice competencies. Instead, in both primary care and acute care ambulatory settings, APNs are most appropriately and effectively employed to perform comprehensive patient assessments, make accurate diagnoses, implement treatment protocols (including prescriptive authority where legal), refer appropriately to generalist or specialist physician care, use research findings, serve as an advanced nurse resource to other nurses, precept students, and provide inservice education (Haas and Hackbarth, 1995a).

The Pew Health Profession Commission (1995) has recommended differentiation of practice responsibilities for nurses with associate, baccalaureate, and master's degrees. BSN-prepared nurses are recommended for community-based practice roles and master's degree nurses for advanced practice in primary care and hospital settings, with associate degree nurses focusing on entry-level hospital practice and nursing home practice. However, it is probably unrealistic to expect that associate degree nurses will not be employed in ambulatory care settings, especially given their high proportion in the current ambulatory care workforce. It may be more effective to clearly differentiate RN roles in ambulatory care by educational preparation and continuing learning experiences. Efforts also must be directed at enhancing the preparation of the current workforce for ambulatory care, including retooling those in hospital-based practice, and providing educational and career mobility options for those with less than a BSN degree. Table 7.2 proposes a taxonomy for differentiating the practice roles and responsibilities of RNs in ambulatory and community-based care settings.

TRANSITIONING THE NURSING WORKFORCE TO AMBULATORY CARE

Nurses who have spent most or all of their careers in hospital in-patient practice may be unprepared to deal with the demands and differences in ambulatory care settings. In addition to moving to the new practice environment of ambulatory care, RNs also will be expected to move from direct caregiver roles to those of care managers (Loveridge, 1995).

Substantial retraining and retooling for these new settings and roles will be necessary to convert the current acute care nursing workforce to one with the competencies needed for ambulatory care. Whereas some competencies transfer readily, such as critical thinking and communication skills, others must be developed. A transition period—in some cases as long as six months—may be needed to enable the RN to adapt to the new roles and demands of the ambulatory setting (J. Peacock-Moye, personal communication, March 1996). Working with individuals and groups in ambulatory settings requires adjustment to the differences in the ambulatory care environment, including the strong emphasis on customer-responsive care, rapid pace and patient turnover, more active and direct involvement of patients and families in their care, greater variability in work, necessity for teamwork, and, in some cases, fewer staff and fewer resources.

Table 7.2. Differentiated Practice Roles for RNs in Ambulatory Care.

Associate Degree and Diploma-Prepared RNs

Enabling operations[1,2]

Technical procedures[1,2]

High-tech procedures[1]

Implement and document plan of care/treatment

Patient/family discharge and home care instructions, basic health education

Telephone communications[1]

Delegate care to and supervise less-skilled personnel

BSN-Prepared RNs

Nursing process[1]

Advocacy[1]

Teaching[1]

Train, delegate care to, and supervise less-skilled personnel

Care coordination[1]

Chronic care management of groups or caseload of patients (case management)
   with common chronic illnesses, using established guidelines and protocols; nurse-
   managed clinics for health promotion, disease prevention, and supportive care

Community care, e.g., outreach education and health care services for groups,
   including health

Sources: (1) Hackbarth, D. P., Haas, S. A., Kavanagh, J. A., and Vlasses, F. *Nursing Economic$*, 1995, *13*(2), p. 92 and (2) Haas, S. A., and Hackbarth, D. P. *Nursing Economic$*, 1995, *13*(4), p. 233. Reprinted with permission of the publisher, Janetti Publications, Inc., East Holly Avenue, Box 56, Pitman, NJ 08071–0056 (Phone: 609-256-2300).

Hospital-based RNs prepared at the associate degree or diploma level may be at a particular disadvantage in making the transition to ambulatory care because the knowledge and skills needed for ambulatory care practice are not typically acquired at that level of nursing education. Though they may have gained experience with patient teaching and management functions in their hospital practice, these RNs are likely to need further education in the areas of primary care and community health. A number of options exist for upgrading the education and skills of hospital-based RNs in order to prepare them for ambulatory care practice. These options include but are not limited to the following:

- Specially designed transition programs; for example, combining in-service education with an internship or mentored practice under the guidance of an experienced ambulatory care nurse, as part of the employee's work assignment

- Continuing education programs that focus on the particular skills needed in ambulatory care; for example, telephone triage and counseling, interdisciplinary practice, case management, ethical decision making, continuous improvement, training and supervision of UAPs, and critical pathways–clinical practice guidelines

- RN-to-BSN programs that provide a focused option in ambulatory and community-based care and educate students specifically for ambulatory care roles

- Accelerated RN-to-MSN programs that prepare associate degree and diploma-prepared nurses for advanced practice roles.

As ambulatory services in large hospital systems expand, opportunities for nurses to move from in-patient to ambulatory settings will become increasingly available. Transition programs to prepare hospital-displaced RN employees for new roles in the system's ambulatory care division are needed, and ideally should be provided and financially underwritten by the system. Organizations that value their employees as assets will view this investment in retooling as a benefit to the system and not simply to the individual employee (Flower, 1996).

CHALLENGES FOR NURSING EDUCATION

Significant changes in the nursing workforce have occurred over the last three decades, particularly in size and educational mix, that will affect employment opportunities in ambulatory care. Unfortunately, these changes are not neces-sarily congruent with current and future projections of workforce needs (Pew Health Professions Commission, 1995).

The educational preparation of the current RN workforce in ambulatory care is profiled in Figure 7.2. The percentage of the RN workforce with a baccalaure-ate degree is higher among RNs in ambulatory care than in the RN workforce as a whole (37 percent versus 30 percent). Nevertheless, over half of RNs working in ambulatory settings are prepared at only the diploma or associate degree level. RNs with master's degrees account for only a small percentage (8 percent) of RNs working in ambulatory settings (Moses, 1994, as cited in Hackbarth, Haas, Kavanagh, and Vlasses, 1995).

The U.S. Department of Health and Human Services (1991) predicts that nurs-ing education programs are producing too many associate degree graduates and not enough baccalaureate and master's degree graduates relative to the changing market. This is especially likely to be true for ambulatory and community-based care settings, where nurses will be needed in the future to fill such roles as man-agers, case coordinators, patient educators, and primary care providers. Given that many of the competencies needed for ambulatory care practice are not acquired in associate degree or diploma nursing education programs, significant changes are called for in nursing education to ensure that the future workforce is prepared to

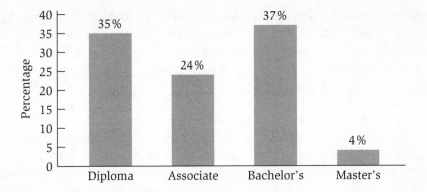

Figure 7.2. RN Educational Preparation in Ambulatory Care.

Source: Hackbarth, D. P., Haas, S. A., Kavanagh, J. A., and Vlasses, F. Reprinted from *Nursing Economic$*, 1995, *13*(2), p. 92. Reprinted with permission of the publisher, Janetti Publications, Inc., East Holly Avenue, Box 56, Pitman, NJ 08071–0056 (Phone: 609–256–2300).

provide care for an expanding ambulatory care population. Such changes must include reconfiguring the mix of educational programs and shifting nursing curricula and learning experiences to ambulatory and community-based settings.

The Pew Health Professions Commission (1995) calls for reducing enrollments in diploma and associate degree programs by 10–20 percent, and expanding advanced nurse practice programs. The nation's nursing schools are responding by initiating or expanding existing programs to prepare nurses for advanced practice roles, especially in primary care. Over 9,000 new advanced practice nurses are expected to enter the health care system in 1996 as a result of increases in enrollments in graduate programs (National League for Nursing, 1995). However, concern has been expressed within the profession and by others that APN education programs are proliferating too rapidly, may be producing more graduates than the market can absorb, are lacking in sufficient numbers of qualified faculty (nurse educators who are themselves appropriately prepared and credentialed for APN roles), and are risking program quality.

To date, enrollment in associate degree programs has dropped only slightly. Diploma programs continue to decline, although some are simply being converted to associate degree programs. Changing the number and type of nursing education programs will not be an easy task to accomplish. Dialogue at state and regional levels must begin to focus on the number, size, and type of nursing education programs that are needed to meet the state's or region's nursing workforce needs.

Clearly, nursing education must be reconfigured and redesigned in order to prepare students for ambulatory practice roles. It will not be sufficient to simply move student learning experiences from hospital to ambulatory settings.

Students must learn how to practice across systems of care, and to shift their focus from providing direct, hands-on care to managing and coordinating care for individuals, families, and populations.

A number of compelling questions highlight the challenges facing nursing education as faculty and programs strive to make the changes are called for: What are the incentives and barriers to preparing students for practice in the community and for population-based care? Are community placement settings available in sufficient numbers and kinds to ensure quality learning experiences for students? To what extent are faculty prepared to teach in a community-based, community-focused health care system? How do state nursing board regulations support or constrain the ability of nursing programs to transform curricula and educate students in nontraditional settings? What are the direct and indirect costs associated with educating students in community-based settings (and who will bear these costs)? What are the implications for faculty: student ratios, faculty teaching workloads, and the use of clinical staff as preceptors and mentors? To what extent are community-based practice sites willing to accept student placements, given the shift to capitated and managed care systems that emphasize cost containment (Bellack, 1995, p. 342)?

The answer to a number of these questions may be the development of partnerships with managed care and integrated delivery systems (Mundt, 1997; Pew Health Professions Commission, 1995). Such alliances could expand the capacity for educating students across a variety of settings, including hospital-based and community-based ambulatory settings. Nursing programs and faculty could partner with these systems to identify or create clinical practice opportunities for students to learn in tandem with appropriately credentialed RN staff in the system. Reciprocally, faculty can provide opportunities for RNs employed in the acute care setting to acquire the knowledge and skills for practice in ambulatory settings through degree-granting, retraining, and continuing education programs.

CONCLUSION

There is little question that the downsizing and restructuring occurring in hospitals will lead to a need for fewer RNs in the acute care inpatient setting. Although the shift to ambulatory services, whether hospital or nonhospital based, has been dramatic over the last decade, its full impact on the nursing workforce has yet to be felt. Nursing employment in ambulatory care settings has grown steadily since 1980, but hospital employment has increased at a proportionately greater rate during the same period of time (Yordy, 1996).

Yordy pointedly notes, "The small proportion of nurses employed in settings other than hospitals means that large proportional increases in these employment opportunities would have to take place in order to absorb even a modest reduction in hospital nursing employment. One can also question whether the educational preparation, experience, and skills of many hospital nurses can be applied in non-hospital settings without substantial retraining. The sources of financing for such training on a large scale are also unclear" (p. 147).

Yordy suggests that even a three- or fourfold increase in employment opportunities for APNs is not likely to be significant enough to accommodate the large numbers of RNs that will be displaced from hospital practice, and in any event, nearly all would require advanced nursing education to assume such roles. Even if sufficient employment opportunities existed, the current nursing education system lacks the capacity and the flexibility to educate large numbers of APNs for ambulatory and community-based practice roles. Further, Yordy notes that because managed care plans (MCPs) have the management structure, resources, and economic incentives to respond to market needs, they may be more likely to create their own innovative approaches to nursing workforce development and training than to accept the profession's model. However, he also points out that partnerships between MCPs and the nursing profession could facilitate educational mobility, assist in removing some of the current barriers to the full scope of advanced nursing practice, and help MCPs compete successfully.

Another force that may affect roles for nurses in ambulatory settings are the grass-roots efforts, identified in Chapter Four, that are taking place across the nation to build healthier communities and respond to community-specific health needs. As community members take a more active role in defining and managing their own health needs, there may be less need and fewer demands for formal community health services provided by health professionals.

In addition, as more individuals and households acquire access to electronic information resources, such as those available on the Internet, opportunities for self-care and self-management of health and minor illness are likely to increase. Ferguson (1994) notes that health care in the information age will encourage individual self-care, self-help networks (both social and electronic), and professionals as facilitators and partners rather than authorities. Nurses are likely to be the health professionals best prepared to respond to the public's desire for a wide variety of health information, validation of their health choices, and "high-tech, high-touch" care. Nurses have gained the public's trust and have demonstrated their ability to effectively and sensitively communicate with and respond to the health needs of patients and their families (Beckham, 1996; O'Neil, 1993; Shugars, O'Neil, and Bader, 1991).

Nurses with the requisite competencies are well positioned to become ambulatory care entrepreneurs, capable of fully managing wellness and chronic illness care, providing telephone advisory services, and serving as consultants and contributors to electronic health information networks. Although such opportunities raise new questions of liability, they also may create new roles for RNs as managers and purveyors of health information. As integrated delivery systems establish electronic bulletin boards or connections to individual health counselors via the Internet, they may employ nurses to fulfill such roles.

In the final analysis, RNs and APNs will ensure their future roles in ambulatory care when they demonstrate their ability to be cost-effective providers who can provide needed services in these settings. Insufficient data are available to document the extent to which RNs and APNs currently are able to provide high-quality care and services at the lowest cost for given patient populations in ambulatory settings. There is, however, substantial evidence that RNs and APNs do have the competencies to meet the complex demands of the ambulatory setting. Despite this evidence they have yet to be utilized to their full capacity in ways that differentiate and capitalize on their respective (associate degree/diploma, baccalaureate, higher degree) capabilities. As hospital-based and freestanding ambulatory services continue to expand and as managed care systems mature, RNs and APNs should find new opportunities for transformed practice roles in ambulatory settings, opportunities that will effectively utilize their cost-effective, comprehensive, and caring skills.

References

American Academy of Nursing. *Managed Care and National Health Care Reform: Nurses Can Make It Work.* Washington, D.C.: American Academy of Nursing, 1993.

American College of Surgeons. *Issues and Perspectives.* Chicago: American College of Surgeons, 1988.

American Hospital Association. *Hospital Statistics, 1981 Edition.* Chicago: American Hospital Association, 1981.

American Hospital Association. *Hospital Statistics, 1990–91 Edition.* Chicago: American Hospital Association, 1990.

American Nurses Association. *Nursing Facts.* Washington, D.C.: American Nurses Association, 1995.

Barger, S. E. "Establishing a Nursing Center: Learning from the Literature and Experiences of Others." *Journal of Professional Nursing,* 1995, *11*(4), 203–212.

Beckham, J. D. "The Engine of Choice." *Healthcare Forum Journal,* 1996, *39*(4), 58–64.

Bednash, G. D. "The Interplay Between the Supply of Physicians and Advanced Practice Nurses." In M. Osterweis, C. J. McLaughlin, H. R. Manasse, and C. L. Hopper (eds.), *The U.S. Health Workforce: Power, Politics, and Policy.* Washington, D.C.: Association of Academic Health Centers, 1996, pp. 209–217.

Bellack, J. P. "Educating for the Community." *Journal of Nursing Education,* 1995, *34*(8), 342–343.

Bey, J. M., McGovern, P. M., and Foley, M. "How Management and Nurses Perceive Occupational Health Nursing." *AAOHN Journal,* 1988, *36*(2), 61–69.

Burgel, B. J. *Innovation at the Work Site: Delivery of Nurse-Managed Primary Health Care Services.* Washington, D.C.: American Nurses Publishing, 1993.

Cohen, R. A. Synopsis of speaker presentations. In *The Proceedings—Crafting Public Protection for the 21st Century: The Role of Nursing Regulation.* Chicago: National Council of State Boards of Nursing, Inc., 1996, pp. 9–16.

Curran, C. R. "An Interview with Linda D'Angelo." *Nursing Economic$,* 1995, *13*(4), 193–196.

Droste, K. (ed.). *Gale Book of Averages.* Detroit: Gale Research, Inc., 1992.

Etheridge, P. E. "A Nursing HMO: Carondolet St. Mary's Experience." *Nursing Management,* 1991, *22*(7), 22–29.

Ferguson, T. *Millenium Whole Earth Catalog.* San Francisco: HarperCollins, 1994.

Finocchio, L. J., and others. *Reforming Health Care Workforce Regulation: Policy Considerations for the 21st Century.* San Francisco: Pew Health Professions Commission, 1995.

Flower, J. "We Are What We Can Learn." *Healthcare Forum Journal,* 1996, *39*(4), 35–41.

Frampton, J., and Wall, S. "Exploring the Use of NPs and PAs in Primary Care." *HMO Practice,* 1994, *8*(4), 165–170.

Fraser, I., Lane, L., Linne, E., and Jones, L. "Ambulatory Care: A Decade of Change in Health Care Delivery." *Journal of Ambulatory Care Management,* 1993, *16*(4), 1–8.

Green, A. H., and Conway-Welch, C. "Negotiating Capitated Rates for Nurse-Managed Clinics." *Nursing Economic$,* 1995, *13*(2), 104–106.

Haas, S. A., and Hackbarth, D. P. "Dimensions of the Staff Nurse Role in Ambulatory Care: Part III—Using Research Data to Design New Models of Nursing Care Delivery." *Nursing Economic$,* 1995a, *13*(4), 230–241.

Haas, S. A., and Hackbarth, D. P. "Dimensions of the Staff Nurse Role in Ambulatory Care: Part IV—Developing Nursing Intensity Measures, Standards, Clinical Ladders, and QI Programs. *Nursing Economic$,* 1995b, *13*(5), 285–294.

Haas, S. A., Hackbarth, D. P., Kavanagh, J. A., and Vlasses, F. "Dimensions of the Staff Nurse Role in Ambulatory Care: Part II—Comparison of Role Dimensions in Four Ambulatory Care Settings." *Nursing Economic$,* 1995, *13*(3), 152–165.

Hackbarth, D. P., Haas, S. A., Kavanagh, J. A., and Vlasses, F. "Dimensions of the Staff Nurse Role in Ambulatory Care: Part I—Methodology and Analysis of Data on Current Staff Practice." *Nursing Economic$,* 1995, *13*(2), 89–98.

Hockey, L. "Community Health Nursing in Crisis?" *Health and Social Care in the Community,* 1995, *3*, 193–197.

Jenkins, M., and Torrisi, D. L. "Nurse Practitioners, Community Nursing Centers, and Contracting for Managed Care." *Journal of the American Academy of Nurse Practitioners,* 1995, *7*(3), 119–123.

Knauth, D. G. "Community Nursing Centers: Removing Impediments to Success." *Nursing Economic$,* 1994, *12*(3), 140–145.

Lamb, G. S. "New Delivery Systems: The Call to Community." Paper presented at the meeting of the American Academy of Nursing on Transformation of the Nursing Workforce, Phoenix, Ariz., Oct. 1994.

Loveridge, C. E. "Preparing the Workforce for Managed Care." *Seminars for Nurse Managers,* 1995, *3*(2), 89–94.

Lusk, S. L., Disch, J. M., and Barkauskas, V. H. "Interest of Major Corporations in Expanded Practice of Occupational Health Nurses." *Research in Nursing and Health,* 1988, *11,* 141–151.

Moreland, B. "Ambulatory Care: An Evolving Health Care Delivery System." *Dimensions in Oncology Nursing,* 1990, *4*(1), 4–6.

Moses, E. B. *The Registered Nurse Population: Findings from the National Sample Survey of Registered Nurses, March 1992.* Rockville, Md.: Division of Nursing, U.S. Bureau of Health Professions, Health Resources and Services Administration, U.S. Department of Health and Human Services, 1994.

Moses, E. B. *The Registered Nurse Population: Findings from the National Sample Survey of Registered Nurses, March 1996.* Rockville, Md.: Division of Nursing, U.S. Bureau of Health Professions, Health Resources and Services Administration, U.S. Department of Health and Human Services, 1997.

Mundt, M. H. "A Model for Clinical Learning Experiences in Integrated Healthcare Networks." *Journal of Nursing Education,* 1997, *36*(7), 309–316.

National League for Nursing. *Nursing's Agenda for Health Care Reform.* Kansas City: American Nurses Publishing, 1991.

National League for Nursing. *Community Nursing Centers: A Promising New Trend in American Health Care.* New York: National League for Nursing, 1992.

National League for Nursing. *A Vision for Nursing Education.* New York: National League for Nursing, 1993.

National League for Nursing. *Nursing Datasource, 1995.* New York: NLN Press, 1995.

Office of Technology Assessment, U.S. Congress. *Nurse Practitioners, Physician Assistants, and Certified Nurse Midwives: A Policy Analysis.* Health Technology Care Study 37. Washington, D.C.: U.S. Government Printing Office, 1986.

O'Neil, E. H. *Health Professions Education for the Future: Schools in Service to the Nation.* San Francisco: Pew Health Professions Commission, 1993.

Passarelli, C. "School Nursing: Trends for the Future." *Journal of School Health,* 1994, *64*(4), 141–149.

Pew Health Professions Commission. *Critical Challenges: Revitalizing the Health Professions for the Twenty-First Century.* San Francisco: UCSF Center for the Health Professions, 1995.

Pew Health Professions Commission Advisory Panel on Health Professions Education and Managed Care. *Health Professions Education and Managed Care: Challenges and Necessary Responses.* San Francisco: Pew Health Professions Commission, 1995.

Phillips, D. L., and Steel, J. E. "Factors Influencing Scope of Practice in Nursing Centers." *Journal of Professional Nursing,* 1994, *10*(2), 84–90.

Shugars, D. A., O'Neil, E. H., and Bader, J. D. *Pew Health Professions Commission Survey of Practitioners' Perceptions of Their Education.* Durham, N.C.: Pew Health Professions Commission, 1991.

SMG Marketing Group. *Freestanding Outpatient Surgery Centers' Directory and Report.* Chicago: SMG Marketing Group, 1994.

Sovie, M. D. "Tailoring Hospitals for Managed Care and Integrated Health Systems." *Nursing Economic$,* 1995, *13*(2), 72–83.

Torrisi, D. L. "Nursing Centers and Managed Care: Collaboration and Contracting." *Nurse Practitioner: American Journal of Primary Health Care,* 1994, *19*(7), 69–71.

Touger, G. N., and Butts, J. "The Workplace: An Innovative and Cost-Effective Practice Site." *Nurse Practitioner,* 1989, *14*(1), 35–42.

U.S. Department of Health and Human Services, National Institute of Occupational Health and Safety. *Costs and Benefits of Occupational Health Nursing.* Washington, D.C.: U.S. Government Printing Office, 1980.

U.S. Department of Health and Human Services. *Health United States 1987.* Washington, D.C.: U.S. Government Printing Office, 1988.

U.S. Department of Health and Human Services. *Health Personnel in the United States: Seventh Report to Congress, 1990.* Washington, D.C.: U.S. Government Printing Office, 1991.

Verran, J. "Delineation of Ambulatory Care Nursing Practice." *Journal of Ambulatory Care Management,* 1981, *4*(2), 1–13.

Waszak, C., and Neidell, S. *School-Based and School-Linked Clinics: Update 1991.* Washington, D.C.: Center for Population Options, 1991.

Weiner, J. P. *Assessing Current and Future US Physician Requirements Based on HMO Staffing Ratios: A Synthesis of New Sources of Data and Forecasts for the Years 2000 and 2020.* Washington, D.C.: U.S. Department of Health and Human Services, Bureau of Health Professions, 1995.

Wunderlich, G. S., Sloan, F. A., and Davis, C. K. (eds.). *Nursing Staff in Hospitals and Nursing Homes: Is It Adequate?* Washington, D.C.: National Academy Press, 1996.

Yates, S. "The Practice of School Nursing: Integration with New Models of Health Service Delivery." *Journal of School Nursing,* 1994, *10*(1), 10–19.

Yordy, K. D. "The Nursing Workforce in a Time of Change." In M. Osterweis, C. J. McLaughlin, H. R. Manasse, and C. L. Hopper (eds.), *The U.S. Health Workforce: Power, Politics, and Policy.* Washington, D.C.: Association of Academic Health Centers, 1996, pp. 141–152.

CHAPTER EIGHT

Community Health Nursing

Exploring New Frontiers
While Reclaiming Old Territory

Marjorie K. Bauman

As the title states, this chapter addresses both the new opportunities and the more traditional pathways for nursing service in community and home-based settings. This exploration focuses on services provided in the home. Nurses working in community settings have a long tradition in the United States. Until the middle of the twentieth century, RNs practicing in the home and community as both health providers and educators were a significant part of the health care system. After 1950, much of this work shifted to the hospital as it emerged as the core element of the health care system. With the passage of Medicaid and Medicare in the mid-1960s, the emphasis on home health returned, but shifted from its earlier community base to a focus on individual services. This infusion of new providers with increasingly specialized skills has grown at an even more rapid pace with efforts to manage hospital usage. The same market forces that now move health care in general (outlined in Chapter One) are pushing home health from small-scale, not-for-profit enterprise to a large corporate industry. Bauman sees an increasing demand for home-based services and moves to control costs, a theme consistent with Harrington's discussion of demand for long-term care in Chapter Six.

She asserts that delivery of home care services requires better understanding and integration with the rest of the system. Other changes in this area will include new technologies, both clinical and communication. Finally, there is need and also some evidence that the community-based work of the visiting nurse will return as a strategy for improving both individual and public health. Bauman concludes that these developments are fostering an increase in aggregate demand for RNs in home-based settings as well as a preference for RNs with advanced skills in clinical practice, supervision of unlicensed personnel, and planning and management of home-based services.

If it is true that history repeats itself, then the future of community health nursing can be more clearly understood by examining its origins and the foundations upon which it has traditionally practiced. As health care evolved over the last hundred-plus years, so too did community-based nursing care.

For purposes of this chapter, *community health nursing* is defined as the delivery of nursing services in the home with the goal of maintaining or improving the health of individuals and families, and, where appropriate, delivering services to individuals within the context of broader strategies for addressing the needs of communities and populations. The terms *community health nursing, community-based nursing services,* and *home-based nursing* will be used interchangeably. Public health nursing practice based in community health centers and other ambulatory care settings were covered in Chapter Seven.

Thus, this chapter will review the evolutionary phases of nursing care provided in the home of the patient and family, beginning with the first nursing agencies founded in the late nineteenth century. The pre-Medicare experience, the impact Medicare and Medicaid have had on traditional home-based community health nursing, and the current trends in this now diverse field will be explored. The author will also analyze trends in the volume of home health services and expenditures for them, as well as the impact of managed care on the practice and utilization of home-based nursing services. From this historical perspective, the author will build the case that community health nursing practice must prepare for new frontiers and new forces while reclaiming some of the traditional roles abandoned soon after implementation of Medicare.

Based on these analyses, the author will explore the emerging roles in home-based nursing practice at the advanced practice, baccalaureate, and associate degree levels. Workforce requirements and trends in both traditional and innovative roles will be examined. Finally, recommendations for basic education, orientation, and ongoing in-service education and certification will be made.

EVOLUTIONARY PHASES OF COMMUNITY HEALTH NURSING PRACTICE

In the United States in the post–Civil War era, most health care provision was based on treating illness and injury and was practiced at home using home remedies passed down from generation to generation. Family members cared for one another, relying on their church and community for support and assistance, consulting the owner of the apothecary or the itinerant healer, and using the neighborhood midwife, often prior to seeking help from the handful of physicians available at the time. People were born at home, recovered from illnesses and injury at home, and died at home.

Meanwhile, many communities were beginning to realize that the increasing urbanization and socioeconomic stratification of the United States were creating health and hygiene problems that extended well beyond the individual and the family. These urban areas usually had a few influential socialites who saw the need to provide care to the poor and homeless, to the sick and injured, and to young mothers and children.

The Early Years

Community health nursing emerged as the major strategy for addressing these ever-increasing concerns. In the late 1800s Lillian Wald began the first formal community health nursing program, located in New York City (Christopher, Reinhard, McConnell, and Mason, 1993). Around the country other agencies also were forming. The Instructive District Nursing Association of Boston was established in 1886 (Doona, 1994); the Visiting Nurse Association of Chicago in 1889 (Moore and Loporek, 1991); and the Instructive District Nursing Association of Columbus, Ohio, in 1898 (Bendekovic and Judson, 1989). Because there were few philanthropic organizations at the time, these nursing associations sold memberships in their organization and solicited charitable contributions from individuals. The association, then, would hire one or two nurses to deliver food, clothing, and health care; to teach sanitation and baby care; and to care for the ill and injured at home (Doona, 1994). The home visiting nurse needed to "have a sound body, a well-trained intellect, and a high-minded self-sacrificing spirit" (p. 89) in order to care for individuals with infectious diseases, burns, and skin sores, to name just a few of the challenges facing the pioneers in this emerging field.

In 1912 the National Organization of Public Health Nursing was organized (Kuehnert, 1995). Recognizing the importance of this work, the Rockefeller Foundation appropriated $15,000 to this organization in late 1917. Another significant event in the expansion and development of the traditional public health nurse's role in society was the 1918 influenza pandemic, which caused 20,000,000 deaths worldwide and 850,000 in its third wave alone in the United States. The influenza pandemic was an unprecedented event (Sage, 1995), and public health nurses played an active role in attempting to control its rapid spread. Not surprisingly, the School of Nursing at Yale opened in the early 1920s, with Rockefeller Foundation support to educate public health nurses (Doona, 1994). Unfortunately, by 1929 the Rockefeller Foundation decided to terminate this early funding support for nursing education.

Golden Years

Undoubtedly the prevalence of infectious diseases (such as polio, measles, whooping cough, and scarlet fever) further shifted the focus of the community health nurse from a concentration on the needs of individuals and their families to a broader focus on the general population of an entire community. Public dollars supported health departments, which organized strong divisions of nursing. Beginning in the early 1900s some of these health department nursing divisions joined forces with local visiting nurse associations to form combined public health–visiting nurse agencies (Bendekovic and Judson, 1989), which emphasized their common mission: to improve the health and hygiene of their communities and to prevent the spread of disease through the provision of community-based nursing services. These agencies typically provided such community-based nursing services as maternal and child health programs (antepartum visits, postpartum and newborn visits), well-child and immunization clinics, adult health supervision, mental health supervision, and communicable disease follow-up. Cultural values were respected and social and community networks were utilized (Kuehnert, 1995).

Community-based nursing services extended beyond individual needs. Aggregate needs of communities were identified, and community-based health care planning and interventions were implemented (Kuehnert, 1995). Community health nurses collected and analyzed data to track trends of communicable diseases, infant mortality, complications of pregnancy, and congenital abnormalities.

As community health nursing grew in the United States, the concept of a district nurse emerged, much as it had been practiced in England since the 1850s. The district nurse was often hired to work in the same area in which she lived. Thus, the community gradually identified that nurse as their nurse. To determine what her community might need, the district nurse initiated scientific inquiry (Christopher, Reinhard, McConnell, and Mason, 1993). She would use health care data as well as her knowledge of the family, community, and its cultural values to assess perceived needs and motivations and to establish priorities in health promotion and education. The district nurse would actively casefind, using an individual in the family as an entree to the entire family. One example of such casefinding includes delivering of birth certificates to gain access to homes, or conducting a postpartum and newborn exam to assess other children or to determine the need for family planning counseling. District nurses frequently followed up on communicable disease contacts and school truancy. Through these various efforts, the community health nurse furthered the mission of improving the health of the community.

Prior to 1950 the home was the primary site of medical treatments (O'Donnell and Sampson, 1994). As a consequence, the district nurse addressed the full range of health concerns and problems. It was a time of low-tech, high-touch, long-term relationships with individuals and their families from generation to generation. From birth to death, the residents in that community would have their home care needs met by their visiting nurse. During what many consider to be the golden years of visiting nursing (pre-1950), one nurse in each district did it all.

EXTERNAL FORCES ON COMMUNITY HEALTH NURSING PRACTICE

Many external forces shaped community health nursing practice. Just as the 1918 influenza pandemic fueled the growth of traditional public health nursing early in the century, advances in medical science, such as the development of vaccines and antibiotics, in the mid-1900s reduced the incidence of and complications from infectious diseases and decreased the need for prevention and treatment of conditions traditionally within the purview of public health nursing. Furthermore, the establishment of Medicare and Medicaid in 1965 fundamentally altered reimbursement for home-based services.

Medicare and Medicaid

Care of the ill at home expanded rapidly after the enactment of Medicare and Medicaid, slowing the shift of care from home to hospital that had begun around 1950 (O'Donnell and Sampson, 1994). Prior to 1965 there were just over 1,000 community health agencies in the United States. From 1967 to 1980 the number of Medicare-certified home health agencies nearly doubled, from 1,753 to 2,924 (National Association for Home Care, 1995). However, Medicare coverage for home health services had important limitations. Although Medicare provided health insurance to more elderly and disabled individuals, it also imposed restrictions to its use. Medicare mandated that home health patients be homebound, have potential to be rehabilitated, and require skilled care that had to be of an intermittent nature. Initially, the Medicare benefit was restricted to one hundred visits under Medicare Part A and required a three-day prior hospital stay. For patients who exceeded the hundred-visit limit or had no prior hospital stay, visits were paid under the Medicare Part B benefit, which required a deductible and patient copay. In addition, Medicare beneficiaries could receive coverage only for home care services ordered by a physician.

Enacted simultaneously with Medicare, Medicaid provided coverage for home health services for low-income persons. Some states adopted Medicaid eligibility criteria that were less restrictive than the Medicare criteria. Under Medicaid the patient had to be homebound and in need of a skilled service, but the condition could be often more chronic in nature. Local tax-supported home visiting programs for low-income women and children and those with short-term disabilities began to disappear.

The Impact on Traditional Public Health Nursing Practice

The impact of Medicare and Medicaid on traditional public health nursing was swift and dramatic. The focus of home-based nursing practice shifted from the needs of the community to the needs of the individual. Suddenly, care was to be provided only under orders signed by a physician, thereby shifting community nursing practice from a nursing model to a medical model, from prevention and health promotion to recovery and rehabilitation from an acute episode of an illness, and from aggregate health planning and intervention to individual case management. The impact of Medicare, and Medicaid to a somewhat lesser degree, on traditional public health nursing cannot be overemphasized.

Now that there were two major third-party payers (Medicare and Medicaid), local tax dollars and donations (from individuals and groups in the community) for prevention and chronic care services, such as adult health supervision and mental health counseling, began to diminish (Kuehnert, 1995). Medicare imposed significant regulation on home health agencies, defining how charges were to be determined and administered, what costs were allowable or nonallowable, and what services were covered. Payment would be made for care to a patient with a particular acute condition, and not to his or her family. Care was to be intermittent and time-limited with a focus on recovery and rehabilitation from an acute episode.

The impact of Medicare did not end there. Medicare also required a home health agency to directly provide nursing plus one other covered service (such as physical therapy, speech and language pathology, occupational therapy, medical social services, or personal care aide services). Regulations further specified the qualifications for each professional practitioner, and allowed higher charges for these skilled services. The nurse who had previously assisted the patient with everything, with help from the patient's family and friends, soon found herself delegating personal care to an aide, counseling to a social worker, and rehabilitation to one or more therapists.

The patient soon had an army of strangers marching through his or her home. Whereas in the past the community health nurse did it all, assisting families episodically over a long period of time, now the nurse was one of many providers of specialized care to an individual (not the family) for a time-limited acute care need under the supervision of a primary care physician. As more care was provided by this myriad of agency personnel, responsibility shifted from the family to professional and technical staff, thus diminishing the role of family members in caring for one another. This shift coincided with changes in the family structure: two-wage-earner families, increased mobility with resultant decrease in proximity to the extended family, and increased numbers of people living alone due to divorce or death of a spouse.

FROM HIGH TOUCH TO HIGH TECH, FROM GENERALIST TO SPECIALIST

As care at home shifted from primary and secondary prevention to care of acute episodes of illness, community health nursing care was transformed in two major ways. First, the character of community nursing services shifted from "high touch" to "high tech." This trend became most pronounced in the mid-1980s. When Medicare hospital reimbursement switched in 1983 from a pure cost-based system to one based on established fees per diagnostic-related group (DRG) (Geniusz, 1995), the health industry began looking to home health care as a less costly alternative site for patient recovery and treatment. At the same time, portable, relatively user-friendly, medically safe, and often life-sustaining equipment and treatments were developed that could be adapted for use in a noninstitutional setting. Use of blood glucose monitors, oxymeters, apnea monitors, ultrasound, oxygen, ventilators, phototherapy, and infusion pumps became more and more common in the home. As a result, the major component of growth in home-based nursing care during the 1980s was in the area of highly technical treatment modalities for the sick patient at home (Balinsky, 1995).

Infusion therapy is a prime example of the expansion of a high-tech, community-based treatment modality. Table 8.1 depicts this rapid growth in home infusion therapy.

Infusion therapy is most commonly used for patients with acquired immune deficiency syndrome (AIDS), cancer, pneumonia, complications of pregnancy,

Table 8.1. The U.S. Home Care Services Market, 1989–1999 (in Millions of Dollars).

Year	Nursing and Allied Services[1]	Infusion Therapies[2]	Respiratory Therapies[3]	Home Rental Dialysis[4]	Total[5]
1989	$5,907	$1,705	$315	$1,246	$9,444
1991	9,942	2,596	563	2,032	15,613
1993	15,891	4,088	896	3,218	24,858
1995	22,841	6,197	1,258	4,786	36,132
1997	30,183	8,920	1,632	6,768	48,865
1999	37,865	12,441	2,070	8,927	63,000

1. Nursing and Allied Services include skilled nursing, physical therapy, speech pathology, occupational therapy, and homemaker/homecare aides.

2. Infusion Therapies comprise nursing services for administration of antibiotics, chemotherapeutics, hemophilia therapies, nutrition, pain medications, and other drug therapies. They include drugs and solutions but not the cost of infusion pumps.

3. Respiratory Therapies are services provided by respiratory therapists and other home health professionals in combination with equipment, such as apnea monitors, oxygen systems, ventilators, etc. This category does not include the cost of the equipment.

4. Home Rental Dialysis consists of services provided for peritoneal dialysis and hemodialysis. This category does not include the purchase or rental of home dialysis equipment.

5. Totals include other home care services, such as perinatal services, adult day care and sick day child care, ophthalmic services, and phototherapy. This total does not include hospice and home medical equipment.

Note: These estimates are based on government reimbursement figures.

Source: FIND/SVP, Inc. *The Market for Home Care Services.* New York: FIND/SVP, June 1995. This material used with permission.

cellulitis, osteomyelitis, and endocarditis. From 1986 to 1990 the number of home infusion drug therapy (HIDT) recipients increased 600 percent (Balinsky, 1995). In the late 1980s, 250,000 patients received home infusion; in 1993 there were 1.3 million on home infusion; and by the year 2000, it is estimated that 2.2 million patients per year will receive home infusion.

In addition, community health nursing was transformed from a generalist to a specialist enterprise. Community health nursing agencies currently find themselves needing specialists in many disease management areas, including psychiatric nursing, pediatrics (and sometimes subspecialization, in pediatric pulmonology, for example), maternity, nutrition support, respiratory therapy, cardiac rehabilitation, wound-ostomy-continence, diabetes, neurology, orthopedics, oncology, and hospice (O'Donnell and Sampson, 1994). Hospice is an excellent example of the emergence of specialty community health nursing programs. In 1984 there were only thirty-one Medicare-certified home hospice programs, growing to 806 in 1990 and 1,857 in 1995. In 1995 there were 13,141 registered nurses employed by certified hospice agencies, and an additional 1,518 licensed practical nurses working in this specialized field ("NAHC Voices Concern . . . ," 1996).

Today home care patients are visited by a variety of specialists in their field. The positive contribution of this trend is that it certainly brings greater knowledge and skill to the bedside. The downside, however, may be fragmentation of care to the individual, neglect of the psychosocial and aggregate economic impact of illness on the family and other support systems, and lessened opportunity to see that person as part of a larger subset of the population. In today's model, one clinician no longer has the laboratory of the community in which to analyze larger health care trends and ongoing community health needs.

FROM A COTTAGE INDUSTRY TO BIG BUSINESS AND BEYOND

The dramatic changes in health care outlined in Chapter One are clearly manifest in community health care nursing. The cottage industry of the early 1900s, in which small organizations served local markets, is being transformed into a big business in which large firms may begin to dominate state and regional markets (Tweed and Weber, 1996). Mergers, acquisitions, consolidations, vertical integration with health systems, and even hostile takeovers are occurring at a rapid rate.

Several statistics illustrate this trend. In 1967, locally owned and managed visiting nurse associations (VNAs), combined nursing services, and public health nursing departments composed 90 percent of all Medicare-certified home health agencies. Initially, proprietary (for-profit) agencies were barred from participation in the Medicare home care program (Shaughnessy, Schlenker, and Hittle, 1995).

Ownership patterns changed dramatically once this restriction was eased. Twenty years later, VNAs combined nursing services, and public health nursing departments accounted for only 30 percent of Medicare-certified home health agencies. Proprietary agencies (many of which are owned by national chains) comprised 32 percent of certified agencies, and facility-based agencies were 24 percent of the total. By 1996 the distribution had continued further along this path, with VNAs, combined, and public health agencies being only 18 percent of the total certified agencies, and proprietary agencies equaling 46 percent of the total. However, the number of VNA, combined, and public health nursing agencies has remained somewhat stable since the 1960s, suggesting that proprietary home health agencies have absorbed growth in the market for home health services rather than supplanting not-for-profit agencies. The facility-based providers are also becoming an increasingly formidable competitor group, as integrated health care delivery systems increasingly receive capitated or bundled payments for wide ranges of services, including home care (Geniusz, 1995); see Table 8.2.

The shift to big business has created major concerns in the industry. In 1995, 17,561 agencies claimed to be providing home care services. Of those agencies, approximately 50 percent are Medicare-certified home health agencies, 10 percent are Medicare-certified hospice agencies, and a full 40 percent are home care providers that are not certified (National Association for Home Care, 1995). In some states noncertified home care agencies are not required to be licensed or accredited and, therefore, are subject to no external oversight or established standards of practice. Clients and families may not know that noncertified agencies are not regulated in some states and may engage these agencies unwittingly, assuming that the agency has adequately screened, trained, and supervised the employees providing care. It is not uncommon for clients and families to mistake any female employee of such an agency for a nurse or trained nursing assistant. As a result, both the patient and the profession are vulnerable.

It has been said that health care has evolved from the original focus on mission to an emphasis on profit and now back to reconsideration of mission (Tweed and Weber, 1996). In community-based nursing the mission in the 1880s was charitable care to the sick and poor. In the first half of the twentieth century, primary prevention, health promotion, and control of communicable diseases were central to the agency mission. In the 1980s there was an emphasis on the business of health care resulting in a focus on bottom-line profit. In the 1990s agencies are focusing once again on mission as a means of defining the framework around which they design business units. For example, is the mission of the community health agency limited to providing treatment to ill patients at home, or is it to promote the health of a population through community-based service provision? The answer to this critical question will shape the future of community-based nursing care.

Table 8.2. Number of Medicare-Certified Home Care Agencies, by Auspices, 1967–1996.

Year	Freestanding Agencies						Facility-Based Agencies			TOTAL
	VNA	COMB	PUB	PROP	PNP	OTH	HOSP	REHAB	SNF	
1967	549	93	939	0	0	39	133	0	0	1,753
1975	525	46	1,228	47	0	109	273	9	5	2,242
1980	515	63	1,260	186	484	40	359	8	9	2,942
1985	514	59	1,205	1,943	832	4	1,277	20	129	5,983
1990	474	47	985	1,884	710	0	1,486	8	101	5,695
1991	476	41	941	1,970	701	0	1,537	9	105	5,780
1992	530	52	1,083	1,962	637	28	1,623	3	86	6,004
1993	594	46	1,196	2,146	558	41	1,809	1	106	6,497
1994	586	45	1,146	2,892	597	48	2,081	3	123	7,521
1995	575	40	1,182	3,951	667	65	2,470	4	166	9,120
1996	576	34	1,177	4,658	695	58	2,634	4	191	10,027

Source: Health Care Financing Administration, 1996

VNA: Visiting Nurse Associations are freestanding, voluntary, nonprofit organizations governed by a board of directors and usually financed by tax-deductible contributions as well as by earnings.

COMB: Combination agencies are combined government and voluntary agencies. These agencies are sometimes included with counts for VNAs.

PUB: Public agencies are government agencies operated by a state, county, city, or other unit of local government having a major responsibility for preventing disease and for community health education.

PROP: Proprietary agencies are freestanding, for-profit home care agencies.

PNP: Private not-for-profit agencies are freestanding and privately developed, governed, and owned nonprofit home care agencies.

OTH: Other freestanding agencies are agencies that do not fit one of the categories for freestanding agencies listed above.

HOSP: Hospital-based agencies are operating units or departments of a hospital. Agencies that have working arrangements with a hospital, or perhaps are even owned by a hospital but operated as separate entities, are classified as freestanding agencies under one of the categories listed above.

REHAB: Refers to agencies based in rehabilitation facilities.

SNF: Refers to agencies based in skilled nursing facilities.

TRENDS IN DEMAND FOR COMMUNITY HEALTH NURSING SERVICES

Several critical factors will shape future demand for home care services. Medicare is the largest single payer for home-based nursing services.

Medicare

In 1992 Medicare constituted one-third of all home care expenditures (National Association for Home Care, 1995). Other public payers included Medicaid, Older Americans Act, Title XX Block Grants, the Department of Veterans, CHAMPUS, and local community grant programs. In addition to public dollars, other payers include private insurance, managed care organizations, and private out-of-pocket payments. In 1996, 3.8 million Medicare beneficiaries will use the Medicare home care benefit. Two-thirds of these patients are female, two-thirds are over age 75, 80 percent have annual incomes under $15,000 (approximately the poverty line for a family of four) and 25 percent have incomes between 100 and 150 percent of the federal poverty line (Deets, 1995).

Prognosticators predict varying degrees of change in Medicare expenditures for home care, from a slowing of Medicare growth to 6.6 percent per year by the year 2005 (from current rates of 10–14 percent) (National Association for Home Care, 1995), to a sustained growth of 10.5 percent annually through 1999 (Schlenker, Shaughnessy, and Crisler, 1995). The Congressional Budget Office predicts that home care expenditures will quadruple between 1993 and 2000 (Lumsdon, 1994). Table 8.3 reflects the Health Care Financing Administration's most recent analysis of Medicare home care growth.

Impact of the Aging Population

As discussed in Chapter Three, the aging of the U.S. population has a major impact on future demand for health care services. This trend will have an especially large effect on demand for home care because the greatest predictors for the need for home care services are age and functional disability. Currently, 3.5 million U.S. residents are over the age of eighty-five, and their number is expected to grow to 24 million by the year 2040 (Campion, 1994). The top diagnoses of Medicare beneficiaries discharged from hospital to home care include diseases and conditions that result in serious limitations in functional status: stroke, chronic airway obstruction, heart failure, major joint procedures, and other hip and femur procedures.

If these predictions hold true, home health care will continue to be a growth industry, and home health nursing will grow in importance. Although the rate of growth in Medicare and Medicaid home health expenditures will decrease as a result of implementation of a Medicare prospective payment mechanism and

Table 8.3. Medicare Home Health: Visits, Clients, and Incurred Expenditures.

Calendar Year	Visits (thousands)	Clients (thousands)	$ Incurred (millions)	Visits/ Clients	$$$/ Visit
1990	37,906	1,940	$2,104	19.5	$55.51
1993	169,377	2,868	10,269	59.1	60.63
1996	278,761	3,855	18,141	72.3	65.08
1999	340,357	4,425	25,097	76.9	73.74
2002	381,746	4,820	31,704	79.2	83.05
2005	412,583	5,140	38,549	80.3	93.43

Source: Health Care Financing Administration Press Office, 1997

Medicaid capitated payment systems, there will be increased numbers of persons needing home care services. In addition, there will be increased use of home care and hospice by nongovernmental payers.

Impact of Managed Care

As noted in Chapter One, during the 1990s managed care emerged as the dominant model for the organization and financing of health care services. According to the Health Care Financing Administration, as of January 1, 1997, nearly five million Medicare beneficiaries were enrolled in managed care organizations (MCOs), accounting for 13 percent of all Medicare beneficiaries. Although voluntary, enrollment of Medicare beneficiaries in MCOs increased 108 percent between 1993 and 1997 (Health Care Financing Administration Press Office, 1997).

Managed care plans play an even greater role in serving Medicaid beneficiaries. HCFA reports that eleven million Medicaid beneficiaries were enrolled in such plans as of June 30, 1996, accounting for 35 percent of all Medicaid beneficiaries. Enrollment of Medicaid beneficiaries in managed care plans increased by more than 170 percent between 1993 and 1996 (Health Care Financing Administration Press Office, 1997). Forty-eight states enroll beneficiaries in some form of managed care. States vary in their enrollment levels and in the extent to which Medicaid recipients have a choice in receiving care from an MCO. Only twenty-five states have enrolled in MCOs those Medicaid beneficiaries most likely to need significant home-based services (for example, physically disabled persons, persons with AIDS), but others are considering expanding MCO enrollment to cover these populations (National Academy for State Health Policy, 1997).

The dramatic growth of home care reflects several of the major trends in health care reviewed by O'Neil in Chapter One. As Lumsdon has observed, "Growth in managed care, advances in technology, and market-driven delivery innovations are converging to push home care to the front of the continuum of care" (1994, p. 45).

In this newly emerging environment of managing lives across the continuum, many skills of the traditional public health nurse should be in greater demand: aggregate analyses of health problems of particular populations, health education for families and individuals, casefinding and health promotion, and disease prevention techniques. But will they? Will the generalist home health nurse reemerge, making independent judgments regarding needs and performing a full range of health intervention functions (for example: personal care, education, counseling) on any given visit to a patient at home? Or will he or she merely follow the orders of not only the physician (who may have a financial incentive to minimize utilization of other providers) but also of the third-party payer's case manager?

Some believe there will be a major paradigm shift away from the acute care model to chronic care (Pawlson, 1994) and health promotion models. In the acute care model, an illness is an isolated incident with a single-agent cause and an intervention targeted at that single cause. With this approach the patient is often in a passive role during treatment for the short-term problem. For example, a patient who is HIV positive or has chronic airway obstruction and experiences multiple occurrences of pneumonia is treated as having an isolated event with a single recent cause. In contrast, in a chronic illness model each incident of pneumonia would be handled within the context of the chronic illness process of HIV or chronic airway obstruction, with treatment focused not only on the pneumonia but also on prevention of future incidents by improving underlying conditions, such as nutritional status. Risk factors and patient response (for example: compliance and depression) would be explored. In the chronic care model, illnesses would be viewed longitudinally rather than episodically, with the patient in a more active role and clinicians addressing the psychosocial adjustment to the chronic illness at the same time as the acute episode is being treated (Pawlson, 1994). All levels of prevention (that is, primary, secondary, tertiary) would become increasingly important.

Implementation of the chronic care model will foster expansion of community-based nursing practice. Strong community health nursing generalists will be complemented with more nursing specialists plus other disciplines, such as nutrition and clinical pharmacy. Pressures from the managed care industry will force all providers to examine the scope of their practice and to think more creatively about their approach to managing both acute and chronic conditions. For example, as integrated delivery systems focus more attention on prevention and reaching out to patients, community health nursing clinics may become a more commonly used alternative to institutional-based and home-based care.

Also, as the care model shifts from managing quality and costs of acute episodes of care to improving health status and managing expenditures over time and across providers, the philosophy of care delivery will undoubtedly shift. Some home care agencies will use the approach of hiring the lowest-cost health care provider, thus increasing the utilization of licensed practical nurses, aides, and homemakers and decreasing the use of professional clinical staff. Other agencies will take the alternate approach of using more highly skilled multidisciplinary staff, emphasizing prevention, health promotion, patient education, and compliance, with the goal of improving health status, preventing recurrence, and decreasing total dollars spent over time. When agencies make staffing decisions, the question will be asked: Is it less expensive in the long run to have a licensed professional educate the patient on how to manage his or her own personal care rather than provide directly the personal care aide service throughout the home health episode?

Organizationally, the emphasis will shift from independent providers to more integrated networks, and from freestanding local providers to multiservice regional providers (Tweed and Weber, 1996). In addressing the needs of the patient, the emphasis of care may shift from a clearly defined medical model of treatment for an acute episode to a community health model of improving the overall health status of the patient and family. And taken more broadly, the focus of care planning would then shift from an individual care plan to one needed to manage a population within a community or a group of members of a health plan.

Although these are strong arguments for embracing a chronic care model, managed care organizations have been slow to embrace this approach. A study completed by Shaughnessy and colleagues concluded that HMOs, relative to the fee-for-service sector, tend to approach some aspects of home health care with a stronger orientation toward a medical model as opposed to the integrated, interdisciplinary, chronic care model of nursing-social-rehabilitation-personal care. This tendency may be due either to a philosophy of avoiding utilization or to a lack of awareness by HMO physicians of the potential value of home care (Shaughnessy, Schlenker, and Hittle, 1994). It may also be due to a lack of understanding or demand on the part of public and private purchasers of care. Regardless of the explanation for these findings, Shaughnessy's study suggests that "those who administer and determine policies for such HMOs might reexamine and consider the increased use of home health care in order to attain improved outcomes and possibly longer run cost reduction" (p. 18).

If one is somewhat more pessimistic about the future of community-based practice, a very different view of the future emerges. What if hospitals faced with downsizing their nursing staff and physician practices faced with ever-decreasing incomes decide that they can provide community-based care with their own staff? The hospitals might argue that there is improved continuity of care for the patient by having the acute care nurse provide follow-up treatments at home. This model, however, furthers the acute care medical model and physician direction of nursing practices. It also only addresses nursing services incidental to medical care, leaving the family with often inadequate support and resources. Such an approach would show little appreciation for community health nursing practice as a true specialty, which requires special assessment and broad-based diagnostic skills.

In the case of the physician practice–based service provision, the patient may receive care at home by a nonnurse. Because the physician can delegate many functions to any level employee, the patient may be managed by a nonlicensed, noncertified person with little or no formal training or supervision. This would cause serious concern if the patient's condition changed in a subtle manner and there was inadequate assessment and intervention.

Impact on Traditional Community Health Nursing

The limitations of managed care are most evident in reports of their impact on public health nursing services. Despite the effects of the Medicare and Medicaid home health benefit, many public health nursing functions were left to health departments. These included antepartum care, postpartum and newborn follow-up, immunizations and communicable disease management, well-child care, and intervention and oversight in cases involving child abuse and neglect. Health departments continued to provide community-based care through clinics, community education, and occasional home visits by public health nurses.

Today, many health departments are beginning to feel the impact of public dollars moving rapidly into managed care organizations. Anecdotal evidence indicates that as funds are bundled or capitated to the acute care provider, responsibility for traditional community health nursing services is shifting away from health departments and their emphasis on prevention, education, and support, and toward an acute care medical model.

Delegation of Traditional Nursing Tasks

Managed care is also generating concern about the delegation of traditional nursing tasks. As more care is shifted from professional providers to family or informal caregivers, new techniques of health assessment, health status monitoring, and patient-family education will be required. If the patient has no family or informal support systems, paid caregivers become a necessity. Payments for such care will certainly further threaten the disposable income of major groups of people, especially those with fixed incomes such as the elderly and the disabled.

As a result of this ever-increasing shift of care from professionals to caregivers in the home, some states (such as Oregon) have already modified their nurse practice acts to allow increased delegation of nursing functions to nonnurse employees (Kane, O'Connor, and Baker, 1995). In a study of nurse delegation in twenty states (Arizona, California, Colorado, Florida, Iowa, Kansas, Maine, Massachusetts, Michigan, Minnesota, Missouri, Nebraska, New Jersey, New York, Ohio, Oklahoma, Oregon, Texas, Washington, and Wisconsin), Kane and colleagues found wide interstate variation as well as intrastate ambiguity and confusion. For example, delegation of injectable medication administration is possible in Oregon, not specified in Colorado, and prohibited in Texas.

Kane and colleagues also emphasize the major difference that exists between assignment and delegation. "Assignment" is merely the general teaching to unlicensed individuals of the techniques of a task, such as administration of noninjectable medications. "Delegation" is the specific teaching of a task to a specific delegate, to be performed on one specific client only. These tasks may include, but are not limited to, suctioning, complex wound care, and administration of injectable medications.

This study also summarizes the arguments for and against formal, expanded delegation of nursing tasks. Proponents maintain that delegation promotes equity among persons who have families and those who do not, because delegation reduces the overall cost of home care, expanding the number of persons to whom home care services can be provided. Delegation also gives nurses greater opportunity to exercise leadership and apply more advanced knowledge and skills.

Critics of delegation, on the other hand, question whether delegation will reduce costs per case. They also fear that home care agencies would use "permission" to delegate without regard to the seriousness of individual clients' needs or the particular skills of individual unlicensed caregivers. Proponents acknowledge these concerns about unlicensed caregivers but believe that quality of care can be improved if nurses are involved in their training and supervision. However, critics question whether nurses receive sufficient education in delegation to delegate tasks safely and appropriately (Kane, O'Connor, and Baker, 1995).

Nurse delegation of care in the unsupervised home setting will be increasingly tempting to cost-conscious care providers, especially those who believe strongly in the acute and episodic care model. These agencies may decrease the number of registered nurses employed relative to less skilled personnel, thus increasing the supervisory responsibility and personal liability of those nurses remaining. Nurse delegation also decreases the impact the nurse can have on patient education and prevention.

In this environment it is incumbent on community-based nursing to be in the forefront of proving the value of the "softer" services of prevention, education, early intervention, family and caregiver support, and informed decision making. Community-based nursing must also document the circumstances under which utilizing registered nurses adds value over that afforded by lower-cost personnel. One can only imagine how health care models would be revolutionized if services were bundled through payments made to a community-based provider (as they are in the Medicare Hospice Benefit to certified home health agencies) rather than to an acute care provider. We must challenge the wisdom of allowing the control of health care dollars to be placed in the hands of the traditionally highest-cost providers. Success in this domain will require community-based providers to demonstrate that capitating them for a full spectrum of medical, prevention, education, and support services will result in better outcomes at equal or reduced costs.

OTHER FORCES SHAPING THE FUTURE HOME CARE ENVIRONMENT

Technology and social trends are also shaping the future of home care. In the future, effective and efficient community health nursing practice may not always occur during a face-to-face encounter between the nurse and the patient. There will be smart telephones that can transmit to the nurse the patient's blood pressure, pulse, and cardiac status; smart toilets will analyze the patient's urine. There will be interactive video surveillance and instruction. There will be home robots, such as Home Assisted Nursing Care (HANC), that will take vital signs, perform an electrocardiogram, test blood glucose and blood gases, assist with medication compliance, monitor patient response, and activate emergency response units. There will be X-rays transmitted real time over cellular modems. Nurses will be able to make a scheduled video visit to a patient's home at one-sixth the price of an in-person visit. On video the nurse can assess patient alertness and neurologic functioning and use an ancillary line to view wounds, lesions, infusion pumps, and the like (Mahmud and LeSage, 1995). These telemedicine tools will be linked to a central station of monitors where they can be visualized around the clock. If video visits become a reality, where will the central station be located—in a home health agency, physician office or home, or acute care setting? The site selection for central stations will determine the locus of responsibility for management of client needs and the framework for care of that patient.

The use of technology is already changing how work gets done. Home health nurses have handheld computers with integrated databases linked to other agency providers, primary care physicians, and hospital systems. Staff participate in inservice training on-line or via teleconferencing, and they listen to audio tapes while they drive. Patients also learn from videotapes, viewing self-care techniques at home. Some agencies may soon utilize vans housing hospital-level diagnostic equipment to take diagnosis to patients wherever they may be.

All these changes are occurring while the home health agency's target population lives primarily in urban areas with increased criminal and drug activity. Many home health agencies are already spending significant dollars on armed escorts and staff uniforms, while others have redlined certain areas within which clinical staff are prohibited from providing much needed care to already marginalized populations.

An additional challenge is caring for a culturally diverse patient population that expects similar diversity in staff who come into their homes. The nonwhite population is expected to be 70 percent of the total growth in the population in the 1990s, with the fastest growing minorities being Asian and Hispanic. Cultural diversity challenges agency staff to be aware of special dietary practices and acceptable social distance, touching, volume of voice, gestures, and eye contact, to name just a few cultural characteristics (Mitchell, 1995).

The challenge for home care is to provide the highest quality care at the lowest price, efficiently managing episodes of illness without abandoning a patient in need. As an outgrowth of these types of pressures, management of risk, utilization, and outcomes may become a growing field of specialization.

NEW FRONTIERS FOR COMMUNITY HEALTH NURSING

As more health care, both treatment and prevention, moves to the community setting, public health and home health nurses should not only reclaim the traditional territory of the early days of visiting nurses and health department nurses but also discover new opportunities for independent practice and specialization. As independent practitioners they can be self-employed as case managers, selling services to law firms and families who need assistance with brokering services of multiple providers. They can be parish nurses for church communities. They can establish joint practices in community health nursing clinics, performing general public health nursing and nurse practitioner functions.

As employees of a home-based care provider, community health nurses will have a variety of roles from direct patient care giver and case manager (for the provider *or* the payer) to chief executive officer of local, regional, national, and even international home health companies. The opportunities are endless!

Within the traditional home health agency provider model, many nurses will find opportunities to work under a professional practice model in self-directed work teams, often organized around a particular specialty. For example, a cardiac home care nurse will develop an acute cardiac treatment and rehabilitation program and work directly with specific physician and surgeon practice groups to more effectively manage their cardiac patients at home, or with payers to prevent serious cardiac conditions from developing within their members.

Nurse managers will evolve from positions of planning, organizing, and directing work, where there is emphasis on documentation review, productivity standards, and case review, to broader roles in quality outcomes analysis and utilization management, as well as program development, patient and staff education, strategic planning, marketing, and profit-loss analysis (Michaels, 1994).

WORKFORCE PREDICTIONS IN COMMUNITY-BASED NURSING

As noted in Chapters Two and Three, nursing employment opportunities are increasing more rapidly in home care than in any other health care setting. Experts predict employment in home care will increase by more than 500,000 jobs, or 128 percent, between 1992 and 2005. This rate of job growth far exceeds a projected growth in hospital employment of 30 percent and total health services employment of 43 percent ("Industry Leadership . . . ," 1995). As mentioned in an earlier section, many agencies will hire large numbers of lower-paid personnel (for example, licensed practical and vocational nurses, aides, and assistants) who will then work in conjunction with a disproportionately lower number of highly skilled (RN) case managers.

Although care may shift to lower-paid personnel, the need for registered nurses is expected to increase at all levels, including staff, clinical specialty, and management. The focus of practice may vary based on the level of educational preparation of the individual and the organizational role of the RN. There will be pressure to have more cross-trained clinicians (for example, rehabilitation nurses) and less departmental, discipline-specific delineations of tasks (Stern and Tidd, 1994). If one assumes an increased emphasis on specialty needs of acutely ill patients cared for at home and an equally high emphasis on managing a population of patients as a whole, the primary focus of practice of each level of nursing can be viewed on a continuum from an individual and family focus to a community-wide patient population focus.

The model of nurse delegation suggests home care agencies may utilize increased numbers of licensed practical and vocational nurses for long-term technical nursing care, such as private duty nursing in the home. Some community home health agencies already are beginning to develop a nursing partner practice where an RN partners with an LPN or LVN on most routine cases. In this partnership the RN opens the case and oversees the follow-up care that is performed primarily by the LPN or LVN.

The associate degree nurse (ADN) may be the category of nurse with the least growth, especially if the ADN is on the same pay scale as the baccalaureate prepared nurse (BSN). Unless nursing develops the professional versus technical RN delineation with distinct pay rates and job responsibilities, most home health agencies will choose to hire the BSN, who has more preparation in prevention, health education, and promotion, and who has extended practice capabilities. If the ADN is utilized at the lower-paid technical nurse level, then the LPN or LVN will be the low-growth category. Such choices would be consistent with observations about nurse staffing trends in hospitals and ambulatory sites that Fralic and Bellack make in Chapters Five and Seven, respectively.

EDUCATIONAL REQUIREMENTS
FOR COMMUNITY-BASED NURSING

As the need for traditional public health nursing skills becomes increasingly important and valued, BSN preparation will become essential. The basic curriculum needs to include approaches to health promotion, disease prevention, adjustment to disability and chronic illnesses, and health assessment and education not only at an individual level, but also family and community levels. Knowledge of prevention, development of health-enhancing behaviors, treatment compliance techniques, and analysis of cost-effective alternative treatment options will also be critical.

These basic community health nursing functions cannot be learned on the job nor through experience in other health care settings, but must be part of one's academic preparation with an emphasis on community-based practice as a bona fide specialty area (much as medicine has done with the specialty of family practice). Community-based nursing preparation cannot be an add-on to the ADN-diploma programs without squeezing out other important subjects or significantly lengthening the coursework. In addition, clinical practicums in community health nursing that prepare the nurse for real-life experiences must take place within home care provider organizations rather than be a friendly home visit to a patient seen in an acute care rotation.

Clinical Nurse Specialists

Although there will be a demand for generalist community health nurses, the significant growth will be in specialty areas addressing the needs of patient populations with specific disease processes—for example, cardiac, chronic airway disease, diabetes, rehabilitation, and subspecialty areas of pediatric nursing (Tweed and Weber, 1996). The role of the master's prepared clinical nurse specialist will become increasingly important in these disease management areas, where the greatest potential for health enhancement and cost savings can be realized. For example, if a highly experienced (and highly paid) wound-ostomy-continence nurse specialist can demonstrate cost savings to an agency by decreasing supply costs as well as the need to do frequent visits to patients, the agency will utilize these services. If an agency establishes an acute cardiac home care program in which special skills are needed to safely manage patients at home, the agency will employ a specialist themselves or share a cardiac expert with other agencies within its network. Master's prepared community health nurse specialists will be used to develop critical pathways and disease management programs, measure patient outcomes and health status trends, design effective patient education materials, analyze cost-effective treatment alternatives, and act as a consultant for staff. They will personally handle the most complex cases and will be on call to triage problems of a complex and unstable patient population.

The current master's curricula for clinical nurse specialists may not be adequate to meet the future needs of community-based practice. Elements of the nurse practitioner training programs, such as an emphasis on strong physical assessment and diagnostic skills, independent decision making, and preparation for prescriptive authority may need to be added to the curriculum in order to prepare the clinical nurse specialist for the level of independence required in home-based practice settings. Effective community-based nursing practice will require clinical nurse specialists who can integrate these direct patient care skills with the patient teaching, program planning, and case management skills traditionally emphasized in clinical nurse specialist education.

Nurse Management

The master's prepared nurse manager will analyze customer needs (the customer being the patient, physician, payer, community, or integrated health system); develop a strategic plan to position the agency for the future; lead the organization through constant and often chaotic change; and establish effective cost, quality, and risk management monitors to analyze the outcomes of particular approaches.

Because home health care is a multidisciplinary practice setting, a master's degree in nursing administration is generally too limited in scope and focus to provide effective preparation for managerial roles in the home health industry. The best preparation for nursing management in home health care depends somewhat on one's area of emphasis. If the master's prepared nurse is primarily interested in frontline clinical services management, a master's in community health nursing, clinical specialty practice, or public health would be most appropriate. If the nurse is interested in ultimately administering a home health agency, a master's degree in home health administration or health services administration would be more applicable. Additional coursework in epidemiology, health care finance, and marketing will be very useful to the home care administrator of the future.

CHALLENGES FOR NURSING

These ever-changing times present special challenges to educators and employers of nurses.

Retraining Institution-Based Nurses

As acute care facilities downsize, there are more experienced, institution-based nurses seeking employment in home health care and other community-based practice settings. This provides both opportunities for creative staffing patterns and increased demand for retraining. To minimize the impact of displacement of highly skilled and often specialized nurses, some integrated delivery systems are looking for creative ways to share staff. For example, hospitals and home health agencies are partnering together by sharing staff in specialty areas, such as oncology, psychiatry, substance abuse, and pediatrics, where continuity of care is especially beneficial. These nurses, many of whom would otherwise be laid off, are trained in home health care nursing and work part-time doing inpatient nursing and part-time in home health care, seeing many of the same patients in both settings. They need on-the-job training in the specialty practice of home health nursing, including the increased physical assessment skills, not to mention map-reading skills, self-defense techniques, infection control in often substandard settings, nursing bag technique, patient compliance methods, and overall adjustment to the world where the patient makes his or her own decisions.

Strategies for Preparing New Graduates for Practice

With fewer hospital positions available to new nursing graduates, home health agencies are being pressured to rethink their traditional practice of requiring at least one year of acute, general medical, inpatient experience. Two strategies have emerged to bridge the gap between home care agencies' requirements and new graduates' abilities. Some agencies are establishing programs in which an inexperienced BSN graduate works directly under a preceptor for three to six months of a formal residency period (Todor, 1993). These nurses must have had community care theory and practice in their baccalaureate education and have expressed an interest in specializing in community-based nursing. The nurse agrees to work full-time for one full year during this residency program.

In anticipation of increased pressure to place new graduates directly into community practice settings, some baccalaureate nursing programs are developing a home health care track. One such program includes course work and a clinical practicum during the last semester of the senior year. Each week during the entire semester, the student has one hour of didactic and six hours of clinical practice in home health care nursing. Prerequisites for this semester includes gerontologic nursing and community health. During the entire semester, the nursing student is required to manage the care of two home care patients (Long, 1995).

As the health care environment undergoes rapid and often chaotic changes, the people and systems within the industry will be subjected to parallel transformation. It is only through understanding the needs of the community and developing special education and cooperative programs such as these that the home health care industry will be able to keep ahead of the growing demand for this very special kind of nurse—the community health nurse.

CONCLUSION

In order to not only survive but thrive in the future health care environment, the community health nurse (working in either a public health or home health practice model) still will need the sound body, well-trained intellect, high-minded self-sacrificing spirit, and sense of inquiry of the early visiting nurse pioneers. In addition, the nurse will need specialty training and advanced practice skills in highly technical disease management areas, or in organizational system development and informatics. Maintaining an adequate supply of such nurses will require home health agencies to develop innovative partnerships with nursing education and integrated delivery systems.

Change will be the one constant as community health nursing enters the twenty-first century, a theme echoed throughout this book. While analyzing and planning for the needs of groups of patients across the continuum, the community health agency must constantly be alert to the rapidly changing needs of critically ill individual patients. Only those agencies and individual nurses who can successfully adapt to constant change will thrive in the new health care environment.

References

Balinsky, W. "High-Tech Home Care." *Caring*, 1995, *14*(5), 7–9.

Bendekovic, J., and Judson, K. "Birth, Death, and Everything In Between." *Caring*, 1989, *8*(3), 42–47.

Campion, E. W. "The Oldest Old." *New England Journal of Medicine*, 1994, *333*, 18–19.

Christopher, M. A., Reinhard, S., McConnell, K., and Mason, D. "The Community as Partner." *Caring*, 1993, *12*(1), 44–49.

Deets, H. "Home Care in the 21st Century." *Caring*, 1995, *14*(9), 50–51.

Doona, M. E. "Gertrude Weld Peabody: Unsung Patron of Public Health Nursing Education." *Nursing and Health Care*, 1994, *15*(2), 88–94.

FIND/SVP, Inc. *The Market for Home Care Services.* New York: FIND/SVP, June 1995.

Geniusz, G. "Future Trends Affecting the Home Infusing Therapy Industry." *Caring*, 1995, *14*(5), 58–62.

Health Care Financing Administration. Online Survey and Certification Reporting System (OSCAR) database as of Dec. 31, 1996.

Health Care Financing Administration Press Office. *Managed Care in Medicare and Medicaid.* Baltimore: Health Care Financing Administration, U. S. Department of Health and Human Services, Jan. 1997.

"Industry Leadership Forum Recommends Strategies for the Future." *Caring*, 1995, *14*(10), 40–58.

Kane, R. "Expanding the Home Care Concept: Blurring Distinctions Among Home Care, Institutional Care, and Other Long-Term Care Services." *Milbank Quarterly,* 1995, *73*(2), 161–186.

Kane, R., O'Connor, C., and Baker, M. *Delegation of Nursing Activities: Implications for Patterns of Long-Term Care.* Washington, D.C.: American Association of Retired Persons Policy Institute, 1995.

Kuehnert, P. "The Interactive and Organizational Model of Community as Client: A Model for Public Health Nursing Practice." *Public Health Nursing,* 1995, *12*(1), 9–17.

Long, C. "Home Healthcare: The Curriculum Mandate." *Home Healthcare Nurse,* 1995, *13*(6), 46–50.

Lumsdon, K. "No Place Like Home?" *Hospitals and Health Networks,* 1994, *13*(10), 45–52.

Mahmud, K., and LeSage, K. "Telemedicine: A New Idea for Home Care." *Caring,* 1995, *14*(5), 48–50.

Michaels, D. "Home Health Nursing: Towards a Professional Practice Model." *Nursing Management,* 1994, *25*(4), 68–72.

Mitchell, A. "Cultural Diversity: The Future, the Market, and the Rewards." *Caring,* 1995, *14*(12), 44–48.

Moore, P. M., and Loporek, S. S. "The VNA of Chicago Providing New Services for 100 Years." *Caring,* 1991, *9*(1), 52–56.

National Academy for State Health Policy. *Managed Care: A Guide for States.* (3rd ed.) Portland, Maine: National Academy for State Health Policy, 1997.

"NAHC Voices Concern About Two Newly Released OIG Reports on Variation Among Home Care Agencies." *Homecare News,* 1996, *11,* 10–12.

National Association for Home Care. *Basic Statistics About Home Care 1995.* Washington, D.C.: National Association for Home Care, 1995.

O'Donnell, K., and Sampson, E. "Home Health Care: The Pivotal Link in the Creation of a New Health Care Delivery System." *Journal of Health Care Finance,* 1994, *21*(2), 74–86.

Pawlson, L. "Chronic Illness: Implications of a New Paradigm for Health Care." *Journal on Quality Improvement,* 1994, *20*(1), 33–39.

Sage, M. "Pittsburgh Plague—1918: An Oral History." *Home Healthcare Nurse,* 1995, *13*(1), 49–54.

Schlenker, R. E., Shaughnessy, P. W., and Crisler, K. S. "Outcome-Based Continuous Quality Improvement as a Financial Strategy for Home Health Care Agencies." *Journal of Home Health Care Practice,* 1995, *7*(4), 1–15.

Shaughnessy, P. W., Schlenker, R. E., and Hittle, D. F. *A Study of Home Health Care Quality and Cost Under Capitated and Fee-for-Service Payment Systems.* Vol. 1: Summary. Denver: Center for Health Policy Research, 1994.

Shaughnessy, P. W., Schlenker, R. E., and Hittle, D. F. "Case Mix of Home Health Patients Under Capitated and Fee-for-Service Payment." *Health Services Research,* 1995, *30*(1), 79–113.

Stern, E., and Tidd, G. "Health Care Reform's Effect on Home Care: Strategies for Survival." *Medical Interface,* 1994, *14*(5), 85–90.

Todor, N. "A Home Care Nurse Residence Program." *Caring,* 1993, *12*(7), 86–92.

Tweed, S., and Weber, A. "Forecast '96: New Developments in the Forces and Trends Affecting the Future of Home Health Care." *Focus,* Winter 1996.

PART THREE

ENHANCED AND EMERGING ROLES FOR REGISTERED NURSES

CHAPTER NINE

How Is the Role of the Advanced Practice Nurse Changing?

Catherine L. Gilliss
Mary O'Neil Mundinger

With this chapter, the book turns from delivery settings to two critical roles registered nurses are playing in emerging systems: advanced clinical practice and management of clinical services. Gilliss and Mundinger track the dynamic growth of advanced practice nursing in both ambulatory practice in primary care and inpatient settings requiring more intensive patient care management. Once again, the movement to more intensely managed systems of care described in Chapter One is the driving force for change. The willingness of these new delivery systems to adopt new clinical care models has opened practice opportunities to APNs. Gilliss and Mundinger conclude that as APNs increase in number and expand the nature of their practices, they may find themselves on a collision course with physicians, who are feeling their practices constrained by the oversupply of physicians and limits imposed by managed care. The arbiter of this conflict will likely be the managed care entities that may well value physicians and APNs for different reasons and deploy them to serve different purposes. The future of APNs may also be affected by the downsizing of medical residency programs. Physician assistants are compared and contrasted with APNs in terms of scope of practice, education, relationship to physicians, and training. The authors examine the costs of APN education and find it to be more efficient than medical education, but highly dependent on state and federal government funding. Although APNs have made important gains, they could provide even greater service with changes in education and scope of practice.

The roles of APNs are changing rapidly, with two major redirections: increased authority in primary care, and more patient management in the inpatient setting.

APN is a new term that includes nurse practitioners (NPs), clinical nurse specialists (CNSs), nurse anesthetists (CRNAs) and nurse midwives (CNMs). APNs are nurses educated at the graduate level, who practice in expanded roles. Most APNs are certified by the state in which they practice, and many also have achieved national certification. Regulation of APN practice varies considerably across the states. Twenty states currently authorize APN practice without physician supervision or collaboration, and forty-eight authorize some level of prescriptive authority. Medicaid mandates states to directly reimburse pediatric NPs and family NPs; Medicare directly reimburses nurse anesthetists, nurse practitioners, and clinical nurse specialists, regardless of location or practice setting. Private insurance is available to APNs when clients request it from their insurer and state insurance law permits it.

According to the 1996 National Sample Survey of RNs, an estimated 161,711 RNs have been prepared as APNs (Moses, 1997). Their distribution across advanced practice specialties is displayed in Figure 9.1. As the graph shows, nurse practitioners and clinical nurse specialists are by far the largest groups of APNs.

IMPACT OF CHANGES IN THE DELIVERY AND FINANCING OF HEALTH CARE ON DEMAND FOR APNS

Advanced practice nursing is changing in light of the changes in health care financing and delivery outlined in Chapter One. First and perhaps most visible is the move toward managed care, whether in a fully capitated model or a point-of-service model. In all of these arrangements the provider takes on much of the risk that had historically been assumed by the insurer. This changes the provider's incentives from maximizing revenue to containing costs.

Because managed care creates incentives to use the least costly provider to deliver a service, nurses and APNs in particular should become valued providers, at least theoretically. Nurses more often use preventive and health promoting interventions and more often counsel and communicate with patients, especially with regard to health education, community resource use, and mod-

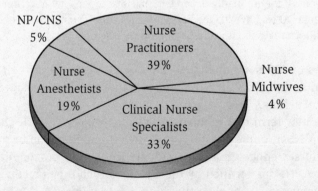

Figure 9.1. Advanced Practice Nurses by Type of Preparation, 1996.

Source: Moses, 1997

ification of personal behaviors and family support to improve health or better manage chronic illness and disability (Mundinger, 1995). These skills are the coin of the realm in the new kingdom of managed care.

But several trends suggest this scenario is by no means a foregone conclusion. First, because nurses have almost always been in an employee relationship at a given health care site rather than in a directly contracted provider relationship with the patient, the costs of nursing services other than following medical orders or institutional policy (taking vital signs and giving medications, for example) have not been calculated or measured the way medical services have been. Second, NPs have been used and evaluated as less expensive substitutes for primary care physicians using the medical model as the standard. Until recently very little attention has been given to the value-added components of NP practice.

Managed care is only one of the changes occurring in the financing and delivery system. Another is the consolidation of insurers into larger organizations across state and regional boundaries. With this horizontal coalescing, the differences between physician and NP services are even less visible. Data on cost, satisfaction, and effectiveness for designated populations, some of which have NP providers, are harder to detect when the insurer being measured is covering such large numbers of persons. A third important difference is the vertical integration of health care, with a health system subsuming the hospital of the past. These health systems tend to provide a wide range of services from intensive care hospital units to day care for the chronically disabled or home care for the frail elderly. Unit differences, as well as caregiver differences, are lost more surely than when care could be measured by site.

The same generic deficit is at work in all three of these configurations. The unique aspects of advanced practice nursing, which were never measured adequately under the fee-for-service system, are nearly invisible in these new systems, and therefore at risk for being undervalued and insufficiently accessed.

Against this backdrop, a growing number of physicians in training are selecting primary care as their career goal. There are a number of reasons for this trend. First, the balance of power between specialists and primary care providers may well shift under a managed care system. Primary care providers will have the power to decide when specialists are used. They will have control over capitated payments and how they are used, and where profit, if any, will reside at the end of the year. This is new authority for a discipline that has long been at the bottom of the totem pole in terms of money and prestige. Second, primary care is where the majority of new jobs will be. As managed care incentives take hold, fewer specialists will be utilized because hospitalizations and referrals for specialty care will be reduced.

Third, medical school students appear to be genuinely interested in the scope and personal connections possible with their patients in the practice of primary care. Many of those now entering the medical profession have different career goals from those entering in the 1980s and early 1990s. The generation of the 1960s has passed on some of its humanistic values to its children, who are now preparing for careers. Fourth, primary care is changing, and it is in itself more interesting. Telemedicine opens collegial consultations and communications to physicians once isolated by geography. New integrated primary care networks make it more likely that physicians will find it intellectually interesting to practice in primary care.

The oversupply of medical specialists means that many are turning to primary care careers or blended primary and specialty care for patients so that they can sustain a full practice. New or existing NP positions are seen as job opportunities for this specialist physician work force. Indeed, in more mature managed care markets such as California the competition has changed already from a price war, in which NPs are cheaper, to outright competition between physicians and NPs for NP jobs at NP salaries.

There is a telling story from California. In 1995 not a single newly minted anesthesia resident could get a full-time job in his or her specialty in that state. One of these anesthesiologists spent hours each week on the freeways in his rusty old car commuting between several hospitals that offered him per diem opportunities to practice. That same year, Columbia University's School of Nursing saw, for the first time, a newly minted certified registered nurse anesthetist (CRNA) secure a full-time job in California at $104,000 per year.

A year later in California, anesthesiologists finishing their residencies were applying for, and getting, CRNA positions in California, now priced at $85,000. In 1996, a CRNA program operated by the University of California at San Francisco suspended admission of students.

Specialists' efforts to reposition themselves as primary care providers will have a mixed impact on the public's health. Generalist training provides a paradigm, a perspective, and a purpose that is focused on the whole patient, a patient with undifferentiated symptoms, a patient who needs a broad inquiry to set things right. Specialists, whether a specialist NP or a specialist physician, are more narrowly focused professionals, geared toward care and cure of a special illness or set of symptoms. In addition, it has been shown that specialists address undifferentiated patients with a bias toward their own specialty (Wennberg and Gittelsohn, 1982). A gastroenterologist, for example, is more likely to perform an endoscopic procedure, whereas a cardiologist would perform an EKG or cardiac catheterization on a patient presenting the same symptoms. The specialist's tendency is of value to persons with chronic illnesses whose new symptoms are often caused or exacerbated by their chronic conditions. However, such a narrow focus thwarts exploration of a full range of diagnostic and treatment options.

This difference is apparent not only in detection methodologies but also in treatment. Physicians, or any professionals for that matter, engage in behaviors where they feel most competent. Whether a specialist redirects the entire practice to primary care or only adopts patients already being seen for particular diseases for primary care services, the inherent specialty bias remains. In addition, the real and valuable skills of the generalist approach have not been inculcated in specialists' practice competencies: primary care is not an uncomplicated subset of specialist medicine.

Perhaps even more crucial, particularly in managed care, is the difference between NP and physician in both primary care and specialist modes. Nurses see the world differently. They use the same scientific method (data, diagnosis, plan, treat, evaluate), obtain the same measurements of biopsychological data, and utilize many of the same interventions. But the perspective, skill mix, and scope of care are different. The focus on active engagement of patient and family as opposed to passive compliance with prescriptions is different, as is the attention to environmental and resource factors in addition to medical symptoms and diagnoses. These differences hold for primary care physicians and specialist NP providers.

What do these trends mean for APNs? NPs and physicians will compete fiercely for jobs throughout the spectrum. NPs pose a competitive threat to both those specialists who are now doing more primary care out of default and to newly minted primary care physicians. Many physicians consider APNs a threat because they have the potential to attract patients who would otherwise receive their primary care from physicians. This competition will affect both experienced NPs and new graduates of NP education programs.

Much of the competition between NPs and physicians will be resolved in price wars. If APNs are viewed as simply cheaper substitutes, when the price differential disappears so will APNs. The public, and indeed the insurers and managed care decision makers, rarely understand that APNs have skills that physicians lack. They know only that APNs have less extensive knowledge of medicine.

If NPs were simply subsets of physicians, hiring physicians for NP jobs would simply be a rational correction in a market in which supply outstrips demand. But this is not the case. Nurses do bring to the patient encounter a different perspective and a value-added set of skills that physicians do not. When a physician takes an NP job at an NP salary, the patient pays less for medical care (assuming the decreased cost is passed on to the patient) but has lost the services and value of an NP. Whereas NPs can substitute for physicians in primary care, physicians cannot substitute for NPs in primary care. But this truism has not been acknowledged in practice or by the insurers who hire or reimburse practitioners. This is doubly injurious in a system that depends on prevention, health promotion, and early detection to avoid high-cost inpatient care.

Research on APNs has been based on more than thirty years of data showing that APNs are a cost-effective substitute for basic primary medical care

(Mundinger, 1995). All or nearly all of these studies focus on the ability of APNs to conduct practice within the medical framework at levels of competence and quality that are indistinguishable from physicians. Until now the focus has not been on practice at the margin, either for physicians or for APNs. For instance, what is the 10–20 percent of primary care that physicians manage that APNs cannot manage? And what is it that APNs provide that is missing in physician care? This last question in particular is what will decide if APNs have a competitive position in managed care.

The incentives in managed care, however, will undoubtedly begin to reveal why APNs *and* physicians are needed in the new system. As hospital care changes and decreases in volume, there will be additional opportunities and demand for APN services. We already know that patient length of stay has radically decreased. It is happening without sufficient patient and family preparation for earlier and shakier hospital discharges. No one convalesces in a hospital anymore, where they can take advantage of health education, learn new and sometimes complex self-care regimes, and come to understand and accept new restrictions or disabilities. Hospital nurses provided these key services, but now patients are out of (if they ever got in) the hospital without these essential post-acute services.

Happily for APNs, the uniqueness in their practice is exactly the set of skills that managed care incentives require. The perspective of wellness—including prevention and promotion and health education; the knowledge of community resources, including home care, public health, and social services; and the focus on the whole patient, as opposed to a focusing on a functional disorder—begins to change the system from one of sequential illness episodes to one of continuous and comprehensive engagement with patients to optimize their health and minimize illness. This wondrous outcome, however, can evolve only if we have the data about differences in practice and evidence of health outcomes that are at least as good at the same or less cost as those achieved by traditional primary care medicine. Otherwise the gold standard of physician practice will prevail, and APNs could become the twentieth-century dinosaurs of health care.

IMPACT OF TRENDS IN GRADUATE MEDICAL EDUCATION ON APN PRACTICE IN HOSPITALS

Surprisingly, as the system evolves hospital settings may be more promising sites for APNs than primary care settings. In academic health centers, most medical care is provided by medical residents rather than by attending physicians. A 1994 Congressional Research Service report (Fuchs, 1994) suggests that the lure of large, urban, primary care networks under managed care will draw physicians from other sites including teaching hospitals. Even in community hospitals that do not provide graduate medical education, physicians are wary of spending too much time managing inpatients for fear of losing more lucrative office visit revenues.

The number of first-year residency positions in some specialties has already declined. For example, between the 1995–96 and 1996–97 academic years, the number of first-year residency positions fell by 30.9 percent in anesthesiology and by 21.8 percent in psychiatry (Dunn and Miller, 1997, p. 752). Although the aggregate number of residents increased slightly during this period, the sharp reductions in first-year positions in certain specialties indicate the presence of increased opportunities for APNs in hospitals that previously relied on residents to provide these specialty services. In addition, significant amounts of education in many specialties are being redirected to ambulatory sites, especially in generalist disciplines.

Two recent developments in Medicare graduate medical education policy are likely to accelerate downsizing of residency programs. In February 1997, the Health Care Financing Administration announced a demonstration project in New York State under which teaching hospitals receive financial incentives to reduce the number of residents they train (Health Care Financing Administration Press Office, 1997). Teaching hospitals participating in the demonstration project must agree either to downsize specialist residency positions by 25 percent or to simultaneously reduce specialist positions by 20 percent and increase generalist positions by 20 percent. In exchange, participating hospitals receive transition funding from Medicare that they can use to develop alternative strategies for providing services previously furnished by residents. The 1997 budget reconciliation legislation (P.L. 105–83) established a similar program of voluntary Medicare incentive payments for teaching hospitals in other states. Though neither the New York demonstration project nor the budget reconciliation legislation mandate that participating teaching hospitals hire APNs to replace residents, the high degree of overlap between APNs' and residents' competencies suggest that such substitution will occur in many teaching hospitals.

Medical residents have a long and distinguished history of providing acute medical care in concert with nurses furnishing support and convalescent care. Now, with the unambiguous future of reduced numbers of medical residents and fewer but sicker hospitalized patients, the obvious professional to provide acute care while attending to safe discharge procedures is the APN. Even if the oversupply of physicians leads to the disappearing of price differentials, the physician just does not have the skill mix or perspective to do this kind of comprehensive care.

The potential crisis resulting from an anticipated loss of residency positions in hospitals could well be staved off by planning for these positions to be filled with APNs (Aiken and Sage, 1992). Even when hospital downsizing is taken into account some substitution will be required to fulfill staffing requirements. Although more traditional voices in nursing will quarrel with the wisdom of the advanced practice nurse functioning in a substitutive role, the practice is not new, as acknowledged earlier. CNMs deliver uncomplicated care to pregnant women and deliver their children; CRNAs substitute for anesthesiologists in uncomplicated situations. NPs have been delivering physician-comparable, if not superior, quality primary care for nearly thirty years. Substitution as house staff officers is the next logical step in the progressive expansion of practice boundaries for the advanced practice nurse.

Data describing the prevalence of use of APNs to fill house staff roles are scarce and tend to focus on short-term costs and revenue streams rather than long-term savings or quality improvement. The development of the concept and curriculum to prepare hospital-based NPs has been described by several authors (Hravnak and others, 1995; Keane and Richmond, 1993). The results of a recent survey by the National Organization of Nurse Practitioner Faculties (Harper and Johnson, 1996) suggest that a growing number of programs are preparing APNs for these roles.

Mezey, Dougherty, Wade, and Mersmann (1994) have reported the results of a survey of New York City area hospitals and schools of nursing to determine current and projected use of APNs in the acute care setting. Consistent with their findings, a number of other authors describe survey findings confirming the increased use of mid-level practitioners (including APNs) as substitute providers for residents in teaching hospitals (Riportella-Muller, Libby, and Kindig, 1995) and in pediatric and neonatal ICUs (DiNicola and others, 1994). Several case reports of the experiences of individual medical centers have been published (Burkholder and Dudjak, 1994; Snyder and others, 1994).

Knickman and others (1992), anticipating a reduction in medical residents and considering the use of mid-level providers as substitutes, conducted a time motion study at two New York City teaching hospitals. Coders identified those activities that had to be completed by physicians and those that did not, and researchers used these activities in two theoretical models, traditional and non-traditional. They determined that, using the assumptions of the traditional model, 50 percent of the identified activities could only be completed by a physician, whereas in the nontraditional model only 20 percent of the activities were physician dependent. Thus, a reasonable shift of responsibility to mid-level practitioners could reduce the need for physicians. Costs were not addressed.

Green and Johnson (1995), in response to plans for New York City area hospitals to reduce first-year resident positions and replace specialists with generalists, completed a cost analysis on replacing residents with mid-level providers. They projected an increased cost to New York City of $242 million annually. Their analysis did not consider the potential benefits of such a change in staffing.

Schulman, Lucchese, and Sullivan (1995) calculated the costs of shifting all neonatal critical care house staff responsibilities to neonatal nurse practitioners over an eighteen-month period. The initial start-up costs were calculated at $441,000 after an offset from a New York State demonstration grant (original total was $722,000). This included education, salaries, staff replacement, and overhead costs. The ongoing costs, which included the loss of Medicare graduate medical education funds (both direct and indirect), were calculated at $1.2 million annually. Care quality was viewed as comparable, and in some instances enhanced by nonphysician practitioners. The authors conclude that nonphysician practitioners are expensive compared to house staff. This is undoubtedly true, given the famously low wages paid to house staff.

The future for APN substitution for medical providers in hospitals is very promising, especially if health care policy is devoid of the answers about differentiated primary care practice. Acute care positions for APNs may grow substantially as the resident work force decreases. As hospitalizations decline and incentives lead to discharge sooner, nurses can make that happen more safely because of their proficiency at patient education, their knowledge of community resources, and their ability to assess the home, family resources, and patient readiness.

ADVANCED PRACTICE NURSE AND PHYSICIAN ASSISTANT: ARE THEY THE SAME?

Given the common practice of grouping physician assistants (PAs) with nurse practitioners (NPs) as "mid-level providers," it is reasonable to ask whether and to what degree utilization of NPs differs from utilization of PAs.

The first PA education program was established at Duke University in 1965. PA education programs originally prepared PAs to assist physicians in providing a wide variety of health care services. Seeking to fill gaps in access to care in rural communities, many early PA programs emphasized primary care (Council on Graduate Medical Education, 1995).

However, incentives for focusing curriculum on primary care were limited. Only in 1985, with the passage of the Health Professions Training Assistance Act (P.L. 99–129), were PA educational programs required to emphasize primary care as a condition of receipt of federal funding. Their eligibility for National Health Service Corps scholarships was first authorized in 1990, with the passage of the National Health Service Corps Revitalization Amendments (P.L. 101–597) (Council on Graduate Medical Education, 1995).

The overall numbers of PAs are fewer than APNs and even the subset of practicing NPs. The American Academy of Physician Assistants (1997) estimates that, as of January 1, 1998, a total of 37,469 persons had been prepared as PAs. Their numbers are much smaller than the estimated 63,191 nurses prepared as NPs (Moses, 1997). These figures represent 14 PAs per 100,000 U.S. population and 24 NPs per 100,000 U.S. population. In comparison, American Medical Association data (1996) indicate a supply of 85 primary care physicians per 100,000 U.S. population in 1995.

As with the primary care physician population, the geographic distribution of PAs and NPs is not uniform. The north central, south, and south central regions of the United States had the lowest ratios of PAs per 100,000 population, and the desert southwest, New England, and northwest regions had the highest ratios. Ratios of PAs per 100,000 population ranged from a low of 0.2 in Mississippi to a high of 24 in Maine (Pew Health Professions Commission, 1995, p. 32). The variation in NP distribution also ranges from lows in the north central, south, and south central regions to highs in the desert southwest, New England, and northwest regions (Pew Health Professions Commission, 1995, p. 34).

Although the distributions generally follow the population, there are a few key states where differences between the availability of NPs and PAs may contribute to the choice of utilization of one over the other. For example, Arkansas reports a high penetration of NPs (28.5 per 100,000 population) and few PAs (1.2 per 100,000 population) (Pew Health Professions Commission, p. 64). One important contributor to an employer's decision to hire a PA or an NP will be the availability of one or the other, which in turn will depend on the practice environments for the two professions in individual states (Sekscenski and others, 1994).

Whether or not the two preparations offer identical service has long been debated. Three factors need to be considered: level of educational preparation, program content, and regulatory oversight.

With respect to level of educational preparation, PA programs were originally organized as certificate programs and did not require a minimum educational prerequisite for admission beyond the high school diploma. Although 64 percent of those entering PA programs in the 1996–97 academic year hold a baccalaureate or graduate degree, 14.4 percent hold only an associate degree, and 21.8 percent have no academic credential beyond a high school diploma (Association of Physician Assistant Programs, 1997). Only 26 percent of PA education programs are at the master's level. This contrasts with NP education, which is almost exclusively at the graduate level, and endorsed as graduate undertaking by the profession (American Nurses Association, 1996; National Organization of Nurse Practitioner Faculties, 1995). One hopes that the completion of a higher degree adds a dimension of problem solving and critical thought to the practitioners, though some sources have questioned this (see Hupcey, 1994).

As described by Gilliam (1994), NPs and PAs face differing licensing and practice regulation issues. PAs are generally regulated by boards of medicine and authorized to practice under the supervision of physicians. NPs and other APNs are generally regulated by a board of nursing and practice on their own licenses. APNs can legally function with greater autonomy than PAs. This, of course, is viewed by nursing as a distinct advantage and raises concern about nurse independence for much of organized medicine.

The vast number of responsibilities created in the emerging systems suggest that there will be room for all providers, and that matching the skills of groups and individuals to the needs of the systems and the clients will be critical to success. The Robert Wood Johnson Foundation is currently supporting an "Education Partners" initiative in which the community-based coeducation of CNMs, NPs, and PAs is one desired outcome. Early reports from these projects suggest that the nursing and PA programs find considerable overlap in the content taught. More challenging is the issue of the uneven levels of educational performance. Some have speculated that this "experiment" may lead to the development of a new generic approach to educating mid-level practitioners for the delivery of primary care. At present, this seems no more logical than assuming that interdisciplinary education of nurses and physicians will result in a generic program for all providers of health care.

TRENDS IN APN EDUCATION

Despite the uncertainty about future demand for APNs, the number of training programs for them has exploded in the last few years, particularly for NPs (Harper and Johnson, 1996). Although some are expansions of high-quality, established curricula, others are first-time efforts to open programs for primary care where quality or scope of training have not yet been externally confirmed.

According to the American Association of Colleges of Nursing (Berlin, Bednash, and Scott, 1997), national enrollments in graduate nursing programs have increased significantly from 1991–92 to 1996–97. Both full-time and part-time enrollments have increased, as have graduations. This growth has been most pronounced among NP education programs. The National Organization of Nurse Practitioner Faculties (Harper and Johnson, 1996) has conducted surveys of NP education programs and reported enrollments for the period 1988–1995. In 1993, 2,812 students were enrolled in NP programs. In 1995, enrollees had jumped 282 percent to 7,926. In the same period, graduates had increased from 1,352 to 3,105 (230 percent) (Harper and Johnson, 1996).

The expanded enrollment and graduation rates of APNs, and of NPs in particular, indicate one or more of the following with regard to employment trends: (1) NP scope of practice is desirable, no matter what the intended postgraduate position; (2) primary care NP positions exist, and enrollees and graduates intend to fill them; (3) primary care NP positions do not exist, and an excess of graduates will provide the workforce for other positions outside of primary care; and (4) expanded employment opportunities in a reformed health care system require advanced preparation.

Barriers to Expansion

Despite the demand for NP education, there are serious barriers to increasing the numbers and capacities of NP education programs. One major impediment to expansion of NP programs is the dearth of experienced, currently practicing faculty who can manage the practice of students while ensuring that their practice is firmly supported by the cognitive requirements.

A second impediment is the scarcity of appropriate clinical training sites. Hospitalized patients gave trainees an almost unlimited opportunity, without time constraints, to learn their craft. In an institutional setting the time spent in learning is almost always an added value to the care of patients. Now, patients seen for learning purposes in primary care sites make themselves available at great personal cost. Most are taking time from work or child care to be seen, and the longer time for a visit, or duplication of history and exam processes, makes it difficult to legitimize the learning process in the same way that hospital training does.

A third impediment is the high cost of APN education, generally borne by the student and educational institution. Whereas both nurses and physicians receive their first professional degrees primarily with personal funds or government or private financial aid, the two professions are radically different in terms of payers for advanced training.

Nurses most often receive their APN training in a master's degree program, enrolling part-time and paying their tuition with money from their full-time jobs, which are usually held concurrently with their part-time education. Nurses usually pursue advanced education after a period of years working in hospital or public health settings. The average age of a nurse in graduate study is the late twenties to early thirties, and the nurse is almost always independent financially from his or her parents. Currently, approximately 28,000 nurses are engaged in educational programs leading to the APN degree and certification (Berlin, Bednash, and Scott, 1997). Annual federal appropriations for graduate nurse education totaled $55.19 million in fiscal year 1996. Much of these monies are for program development, so the actual dollar amount available for student aid is a much lower $19.79 million (U.S. Congress, 1996).

Physician education is entirely different. There are approximately four times as many U.S. physicians in graduate training each year as there are nurses: 100,000 versus 28,000. But the disparity in federal funding is much greater; for fiscal year 1997 Medicare spending for graduate medical education (GME) is projected to total $7.1 billion (The Commonwealth Fund Task Force on Academic Health Centers, 1997, p. 21), and several billion more is provided by other federal programs (Mullan, Rivo, and Politzer, 1993). On a per person basis, there is over thirty-six times more federal money available for graduate education in medicine than for nursing. To take the inequity even further, virtually no physicians spend their own dollars to pay for their graduate education. Medical residents receive stipends, which averaged approximately $35,000 per year in 1995–96 (Association of American Medical Colleges, 1996). Stipends enable residents to complete their education on a full-time basis, an option many APN students cannot afford.

Because of this difference in funding, it is easier to change or redirect graduate medical education than nursing education. Nursing schools generally run on tuition revenues, and if there are paying applicants the schools will provide the programs of choice. In medicine, the federal funds go to hospitals that run the programs; no money means no program, or at least a reduced program. So the federal "levers" for regulating the physician workforce are much stronger than for nursing.

In response to the shift of medical practice from hospital to ambulatory settings, schools of medicine have begun a concerted effort to have Medicare redirect training funds to the site incurring costs rather than only paying hospitals, as has been done in the past. Opportunities for APN education may decline rapidly in the future, because the 1997 budget reconciliation legislation (P.L. 105–83) authorizes the Health Care Financing Administration to reimburse non-hospital sites directly for residents' stipends, faculty salaries, and other direct GME expenses. Primary care sites are already overburdened with medical and APN students, and there will be a strong incentive to close out nursing students, who do not pay for site access, in order to accommodate the influx of medical residents who will bring payment with them for use of the sites.

The desirability of further expanding NP education programs is not yet clear. If, and this is very uncertain, it can be shown that NPs bring a value-added component to primary care, not simply a subset of physician services, then the market should expand easily and fruitfully. If, however, new combinations of providers are quickly established based on the mistaken assumption that NPs are simply medical adjuncts, and if the price differential continues to disappear, then the future is less promising, not only for NPs but for the patients who will be without their enormously valuable services.

Primary Care Versus Specialized Care Training

As discussed in Chapter Two, the majority of RNs continue to be employed in hospitals despite significant increases in RN employment in other settings, especially community–public health settings. (In particular, see Figure 2.2.) Unlike the basic registered nurse workforce, much of the advanced practice workforce is already employed outside of hospitals. In 1992, fully 90 percent of a sample of nationally certified NPs indicated that they were employed in outpatient settings (Washington Consulting Group, 1994). Clinical nurse specialists (CNSs), although still principally employed by hospitals, are completing postgraduate NP programs and expanding the scope of their hospital-based and ambulatory roles (Harper and Johnson, 1996).

Cronenwett (1995) has argued for consistency in the regulation and education of APNs. She notes that although NP practice historically has been associated with primary care, this is no longer the case. Rather, as systems evolve so will the roles of APNs. Therefore their preparation must broadly address the likely needs while sufficiently developing the specialty knowledge required to competently deliver care. Such an approach suggests the need for broad, common areas of knowledge development combined with specialty-based education and practice.

Current educational guidelines and recommendations, such as the American Association of Colleges of Nursing *Essentials* document (1996) and the National Organization of Nurse Practitioner Faculties' *Curriculum Guidelines* (1995) are based on this position. However, they are silent on the question of percentage of specialty prepared APNs in relation to primary care prepared nurses. This silence stands in sharp contrast to medicine, where questions about the balance between generalist and specialist production have dominated workforce policy discussions in recent years.

As with medicine, the case for increasing the numbers of primary care APNs has been made (Pew Health Professions Commission, 1994) and can be well substantiated (Workgroup in Primary Care Workforce Projections, 1995). Further specification, within the broadly defined area of primary care, should be based on population demographics and morbidities. As the Institute of Medicine Committee on U.S. Physician Supply recommended (1996) in relation to growth of the physician workforce, NP (or physician) FTE should be distinguished from NP (or physician) services; the supply of services should be tied to the aggregated, national requirements for care. Salmon (personal communication, 1996) has argued that the versatility of the APN workforce to provide services in many settings and to many patient groups makes support of APN education a particularly good federal investment. Nurses prepared for advanced practice are not setting bound and generally can move with ease among service, education, and research.

One aspect of preparation for advanced practice nursing receiving greater emphasis is the need to incorporate skills for continued lifelong learning. The broadly prepared provider will need to develop new knowledge and expertise as a career matures in order to competently care for populations only minimally addressed in the educational program. If educational programs can prepare primary care providers for beginning practice who are able to continue their learning beyond the formal educational program, then the profession must accept some responsibility to monitor the continued competence of those providers. Mandated continuing education, continued competency demonstration for re-licensure, and monitoring the quality of care actually delivered should be high priorities.

Competencies for Hospital Practice in Roles Formerly Filled by House Staff

As discussed earlier, one major opportunity for growth in advanced practice nursing lies in hospital-based practice in a role formerly filled by house staff. Anytime a new role emerges, advanced practice nursing must ask itself whether current educational standards are adequate to ensure APNs are competent to function in the new role. Given that research on the use of APNs in house staff roles is limited, determining a skill set for implementation of the role appears to be largely speculative. The responsibilities currently assigned to house staff would arguably be carried out more effectively by APNs. In particular, APNs are better prepared to provide care continuity across settings and health education. With one caveat, current preparation for advanced nursing practice is probably close to adequate to support implementation of this role. Graduate programs preparing APNs focus on scientific knowledge, rather than the practical skills that would be required for hospital practice. Although additional skills might be included in the graduate curriculum (such as advanced phlebotomy, sutur-ing, cut downs, advanced X-ray interpretation), this is one area where service and education could provide a better interface thorough coordinated efforts. Procedural learning is often a function of the institutional practices and best left to the service organization. APN education programs should place a higher pri-ority on coordinating service-based learning experiences for students.

THE SCOPE OF ANP PRACTICE: IS IT ADEQUATE?

Recently, the American Nurses Association (ANA) published *Scope and Stan-dards of Advanced Practice Registered Nursing* (1996). This document, developed by the Advanced Practice Registered Nursing Task Force, provides a framework for addressing the issue of further expansion of the scope of advanced practice nursing.

The APN performs many of the functions performed by basic nurses but with preparation at the graduate level practices with greater synthesis of data and complexity of skills and intervention (American Nurses Association, 1996). According to ANA, the mission of advanced practice nursing is to provide expert-quality comprehensive nursing care to clients. Advanced practice is dis-tinguished by autonomy of practice. It is further characterized by an expanded knowledge base, increasing complexity of clinical decision making, and greater skill in managing both organizations and health care environments. APNs are prepared for specialization, expansion, and advancement in practice.

Specialization refers to concentration on one part of the field of nursing. Expansion addresses the acquisition of new skills and knowledge for practice to extend beyond traditional boundaries of nursing practice. Advancement "involves both specialization and expansion and is characterized by the integration of a broad range of theoretical, research-based and experiential knowledge that occurs as part of study and supervised practice at the graduate level" (American Nurses Association, 1996, p. 2). Taken in this context, expansion of practice becomes one dimension of professional advancement, and, as such, expansion of practice can be seen as one essential characteristic of professional vitality and evolution.

The dramatic impact of managed care on health care delivery has been emphasized repeatedly throughout this book. Other documents have described the competencies required for health care clinicians who will practice in managed care settings (Pew Health Professions Commission, 1994). APNs will increasingly be utilized across settings to meet the complex and dynamic needs of clients and will be required to reason and act independently, while communicating and collaborating with others on the health care team. Roles will change as the structures of specific delivery settings change and the number of ancillary personnel available to deliver needed patient care services decreases. APNs will need to be prepared for a broad scope of practice, involving health promotion and protection education, disease management, pain control, systems intervention and community appraisal and intervention, and appropriate tools for evaluation of outcomes.

Recently released documents such as the American Association of Colleges of Nursing's *Essentials of Master's Education for Advanced Practice Nursing* (1996) and the National Organization of Nurse Practitioner Faculties' *Curriculum Guidelines and Program Standards* (1995) provide some evidence of professional acknowledgment of the educational content necessary to instill advanced practice nurses with the needed competencies. Broad preparation for specialty practice that is population based, systems competent, and collaborative, and emphasizes autonomous decision making is clearly described. No significant changes in education are required to prepare advanced practice nurses for a changed health care market. However, two additions are essential for effective practice in the future: APNs need to better understand the economics of the health care delivery system, and they must learn how to measure the value they add to the care delivered.

From a regulatory perspective, advanced nursing practice is hampered by limited scope of responsibilities in some states and a general level of inconsistencies among states. Henderson, Fox-Grage, and Lewis (1995) report that scope of practice for APNs has expanded over the last two decades, as many states have passed legislation or promulgated rules to permit greater responsibility. Although variation continues among them, forty-three states and the District of

Columbia allow prescriptive authority; most states permit independent nurse practice with protocols or referral; and nine states permit completely independent practice. Hospital admitting privileges, most often unregulated and addressed by individual hospitals, have been addressed by legislation in Florida and Oregon. Although Medicaid reimbursement is mandated for RNs, Connecticut, Louisiana, and the District of Columbia do not reimburse APNs. Twenty-five states reimburse APNs at rates equivalent to those paid for physician services, and the remaining twenty-three reimburse APNs at 50 to 99 percent of physician rates. Direct access to APNs in managed care organizations has not been specifically addressed in most states, though some states have enacted statutes permitting APNs to function as "gatekeepers" under Medicaid-managed care. Immunity from civil liability for APNs offering charity care is available in eight states and for those practicing in rural areas in Texas.

Despite the apparently favorable legal climate, Henderson, Fox-Grage, and Lewis (1995) point out that lack of standardization among the states causes confusion and inhibits national unity among APNs. A reduced scope of practice can contribute to a reduction in the numbers of APNs interested to practice in certain jurisdictions (see also Sekscenski and others, 1994; Wilken, 1995). Interpretations of legislation can interfere with the implementation of expansions of scope of practice. Examples include Employee Retirement Income Security Act rules that override state law and conflicting interpretations of statutes, such as Kentucky's Board of Registered Nursing interpreting state law as authorizing prescriptive privilege for APNs while the state's Pharmacy Board prohibits pharmacists from filling those prescriptions (Gilliam, 1994; Safriet, 1994).

The most critical issue in APN scope of practice involves creating similarities among states. One approach to addressing this problem has been initiated by the National Council of State Boards of Nursing, whose 1995 national House of Delegates mandated that the four organizations offering national specialty certification to NPs (American Nurses Credentialing Center, American Academy of Nurse Practitioners, National Certification Corporation, and National Certification Board for Pediatric Nurse Practitioners and Nurses) develop a document reporting the exam requirements and standardization characteristics of all examinations to be used by state boards in reviewing credentials for practice. The long-term goal of this effort is adoption of similar scopes of practice by all states, given the consistent measure of specialty competence.

In a second project, the National Council of State Boards of Nursing and the National Organization of Nurse Practitioner Faculties have been funded by the Bureau of Health Professions' Division of Nursing and the Agency for Health Care Policy Research to develop curriculum guidelines and program standards for the pharmacologic training of family nurse practitioners and related evaluation criteria to be used by member boards to evaluate FNPs for prescribing privileges. This effort is similarly targeted at standardizing training and credentialing.

The project's objective is to assist states in evaluating credentials and ultimately paving the way for scope-of-practice laws than are similar across states.

CONCLUSION

In this chapter we have presented our view that the opportunities for APNs are increasing as a function of role overlap, managed care–driven cost reductions, and recognition of the quality of care that the APN is able to deliver. The interaction of these three factors creates an opportunity for the APN to demonstrate substitutability for other providers, notably physicians. A greater challenge for APNs comes in demonstrating the value they add to health care teams and in the delivery of services to patients. The following conclusions seem warranted:

More advanced practice nurses will be needed, and, because of their malleability, they will find employment in situations and settings in which they were not initially prepared to practice. For instance, many APNs will be working across institutions and settings, following persons with health care problems regardless of their location. Thus APN preparation should not be designed as setting based.

APN scope of practice will continue to evolve and expand, as it has over the last thirty years. Many health care activities traditionally thought of as within the purview of medicine will continue to find their way into nursing practice. This evolution will be influenced by the legislated scope of practice within each of the fifty states. Distribution of APNs across and within states will continue to be influenced by practice climate.

APNs and to some extent the public will continue to experience confusion about the distinctness of the APN role from those of physicians and physician assistants. The APN will be challenged to demonstrate a distinct contribution in the delivery of care and to rationalize the need for preparation at a graduate level.

Thus, we believe the future is bright for APNs. Their success will hinge on their ability to distinguish the unique aspects of APN practice and to document their value to a system increasingly focused on prevention, health promotion, healthier lifestyles, and better use of community health resources. This will require concerted, systematic efforts on the part of clinicians, administrators, and educators.

References

Aiken, L., and Sage, W. "Staffing National Health Care Reform: A Role for Advanced Practice Nurses." *Akron Law Review,* 1992, *26*(2), 187–211.

American Academy of Physician Assistants. *Information Update: Projected Number of PAs in Clinical Practice as of January 1998.* Alexandria, Va.: American Academy of Physician Assistants, 1997.

American Association of Colleges of Nursing. *The Essentials of Master's Education for Advanced Practice Nursing.* Washington, D.C.: American Association of Colleges of Nursing, 1996.

American Medical Association. *Physician Characteristics and Distribution, 1996/97 Edition.* Chicago: American Medical Association, 1996.

American Nurses Association. *Scope and Standards of Advanced Practice Registered Nursing.* Washington, D.C.: American Nurses Association, 1996.

Association of American Medical Colleges. *AAMC Data Book: Statistical Information Related to Medical Education.* Washington, D.C.: Association of American Medical Colleges, 1996.

Association of Physician Assistant Programs. *Thirteenth Annual Report on Physician Assistant Educational Programs in the United States, 1996–1997.* Alexandria, Va.: Association of Physician Assistant Programs, 1997.

Berlin, L. E., Bednash, G. D., and Scott, D. L. *1996–97 Enrollments and Graduations in Baccalaureate and Graduate Programs in Nursing.* Washington, D.C.: American Association of Colleges of Nursing, 1997.

Burkholder, J., and Dudjak, L. "The Mid-Level Practitioner Role: One Medical Center's Experience." *AACN Clinical Issues,* 1994, *5*(3), 369–403.

The Commonwealth Fund Task Force on Academic Health Centers. *Leveling the Playing Field: Financing the Mission of Academic Health Centers.* New York: The Commonwealth Fund, 1997.

Council on Graduate Medical Education. *Physician Assistants in the Health Workforce 1994: Final Report of the Advisory Group on Physician Assistants and the Workforce.* Rockville, Md.: Special Projects Branch, Division of Medicine, U.S. Bureau of Health Professions, U.S. Department of Health and Human Services, 1995.

Cronenwett, L. "Molding the Future of Advanced Practice Nursing." *Nursing Outlook,* 1995, *34*(3), 112–118.

DiNicola, L., and others. "Use of Pediatric Physician Extenders in Pediatrics and Neonatal Intensive Care Units." *Critical Care Medicine,* 1994, *22*(11), 1856–1864.

Dunn, M. R., and Miller, R. S. "U.S. Graduate Medical Education, 1996–1997." *Journal of the American Medical Association,* 1997, *278*(9), 750–754.

Fishman, L. *Medicare Payments with an Education Label: Fundamentals and the Future.* Washington, D.C.: Association of American Medical Colleges, 1996.

Fuchs, B. *Health Care Reform: Managed Competition in Rural Areas.* (CRS Report for Congress 94–336 EPW). Washington, D.C.: Congressional Research Service, 1994.

Gilliam, J. "A Contemporary Analysis of Medicolegal Concerns for Physicians Assistants and Nurse Practitioners." *Legal Medicine,* 1994, 133–180.

Green, B., and Johnson, T. "Replacing Residents with Mid-Level Practitioners: A New York City Area Analysis." *Health Affairs,* 1995, *14*(2), 192–198.

Harper, D., and Johnson, J. *Workforce Policy Project Technical Report: Nurse Practitioner Educational Programs 1988–1995.* Washington, D.C.: National Organization of Nurse Practitioner Faculties, 1996.

Health Care Financing Administration Press Office. "New York Teaching Hospitals Participate in Graduate Medical Education Demonstration." Washington, D.C.: Health Care Financing Administration, U.S. Department of Health and Human Services, Feb. 17, 1997.

Henderson, T., Fox-Grage, W., and Lewis, S. *Scope of Practice and Reimbursement for Advanced Practice Nurses: A State by State Analysis.* Washington, D.C.: Intergovernmental Health Policy Project, George Washington University, 1995.

Hravnak, M., and others. "Acute Care Nurse Practitioner Curriculum: Content and Development Process." *American Journal of Critical Care,* 1995, *4*(3), 179–188.

Hupcey, J. "Graduate Education for Nurse Practitioners: Are Advanced Degrees Needed for Practice?" *Journal of Professional Nursing,* 1994, *10*(8), 350–356.

Institute of Medicine, Committee on the U.S. Physician Supply. *The Nation's Physician Workforce: Options for Balancing Supply and Requirements.* Washington, D.C.: National Academy Press, 1996.

Keane, A., and Richmond, T. "Tertiary Nurse Practitioners." *Image,* 1993, *25*(4), 281–284.

Knickman, J., and others. "The Potential for Using Non-Physicians to Compensate for the Reduced Availability of Residents." *Academic Medicine,* 1992, *429,* 431–435.

Mezey, M., Dougherty, M., Wade, P., and Mersmann, C. "Nurse Practitioners, Certified Nurse Midwives, and Nurse Anesthetists: Changing Care in Acute Care Hospitals in New York City." *Journal of the New York State Nurses Association,* 1994, *25*(4), 13–17.

Moses, E. B. *The Registered Nurse Population: Findings from the National Sample Survey of Registered Nurses, March 1996.* Rockville, Md.: Division of Nursing, U.S. Bureau of Health Professions, Health Resources and Services Administration, Public Health Service, U.S. Department of Health and Human Services, 1997.

Mullan, F., Rivo, M. L., and Politzer, R. M. "Doctors, Dollars, and Determination: Making Physician Workforce-Policy." *Health Affairs,* Sept. 1993, pp. 138–149.

Mundinger, M. "Advanced Practice Nursing—Good Medicine for Physicians?" *New England Journal of Medicine,* 1995, *15*(1), 28–33.

National Organization of Nurse Practitioner Faculties. *Curriculum Guidelines and Program Standards, Second Edition.* Washington, D.C.: National Organization of Nurse Practitioner Faculties, 1995.

Pew Health Professions Commission. *Primary Care Workforce 2000: Federal Policy Paper.* San Francisco: UCSF Center for the Health Professions, 1994.

Pew Health Professions Commission. *State Health Personnel Handbook: Data for the Fifty States.* San Francisco: UCSF Center for the Health Professions, 1995.

Riportella-Muller, R., Libby, D., and Kindig, D. "The Substitution of Physicians Assistants and Nurse Practitioners for Physician Residents in Teaching Hospitals." *Health Affairs,* 1995, *14*(2), 181–191.

Safriet, B. "Impediments to Progress in Health Care Workforce Policy: License and Practice Laws." *Inquiry,* 1994, *31,* 310–317.

Schulman, M., Lucchese, K., and Sullivan, A. "Transition from House Staff to Non-Physician Neonatal Intensive Care Providers: Cost, Impact on Revenues and Quality of Care." *American Journal of Perinatology,* 1995, *12*(6), 442–446.

Sekscenski, E. "Physicians Assistants." In *1993 Health Personnel in the United States: Ninth Report to Congress.* Rockville, Md.: U.S. Bureau of Health Professions, U.S. Department of Health and Human Services, 1993.

Sekscenski, E., and others. "State Practice Environments and the Supply of Physicians Assistants, Nurse Practitioners and Certified Nurse Midwives." *New England Journal of Medicine,* 1994, *331*(19), 1266–1271.

Snyder, J., and others. "Trial of Nurse Practitioners in the ICU." *New Horizons,* 1994, *2*(3), 296–304.

U.S. Congress. *Fiscal Year 1996 Omnibus Consolidated Recisions and Appropriations Act,* Public Law 104–134.

Washington Consulting Group. *Survey of Certified Nurse Practitioners and Clinical Nurse Specialists: December 1992.* Prepared under contract with Division of Nursing, U.S. Bureau of Health Professions, U.S. Department of Health and Human Services. Washington, D.C., 1994.

Wennberg, J., and Gittelsohn, A. "Variations in Medical Care Among Small Areas." *Scientific American,* 1982, *246,* 120–134.

Wilken, M. "State Regulatory Board Structure, Regulations, and Nurse Practitioner Availability." *Nurse Practitioner,* 1995, *20*(10), 68–74.

Workgroup on Primary Care Workforce Projections. *Final Report.* Rockville, Md.: Bureau of Health Professions, Health Resources and Services Administration, U.S. Department of Health and Human Services, 1995.

CHAPTER TEN

From Case Management to Medical Care Management

Implications for Nursing Education

Barry R. Greene
Debra L. Kelsey

This chapter examines the traditional role of the registered nurse as case manager and explores how that role will change in the context of the managed systems of care outlined in Chapter One and described in greater depth in Chapter Four. As management of medical services becomes increasingly important, these systems will demand that some professionals exercise leadership in this area. Nursing professionals already have a significant amount of training and experience in case management and could be directed to expand their skill base to encompass the larger role of care manager needed by the new health systems. The chapter closes with suggestions on how the gap between RNs' current skills and those required for medical care management can be filled. The authors conclude that improving an RN's skills in analyzing and conducting health services research will be essential to narrowing this gap.

The dramatic changes in the health care industry described in Chapter One and throughout this book are creating intense pressure to reduce costs, maintain revenues, and improve quality. These pressures are increasingly compelling health care providers to accept more accountability for lowering costs and improving quality. This emphasis has led to more active involvement on the part of health professionals in constructing measurement mechanisms that can demonstrate accountability and capacity to meet consumer needs. Figure 10.1 depicts the activities and processes of shared accountability. These activities involve learning and applying the tools of systems analysis and quality management. They also encompass new ways of thinking about the measurement of health care processes and inputs.

Establishing a clinically integrated health care system has become a predominant strategy for improving accountability. At the core of this strategy, care management programs provide for continuity of care across the continuum of services and clinical settings. Care management encompasses planning, assessment, and

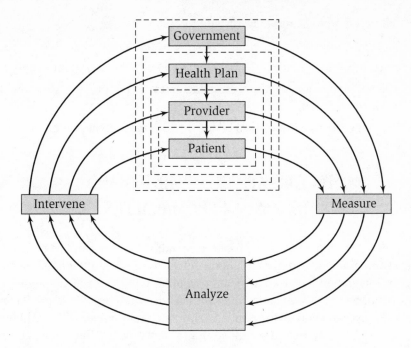

Figure 10.1. Medical Management and Shared Accountabilities Model.
Source: Strategic Consulting Services, 1995.

coordination of health services for the population managed by a delivery system. Some care management activities focus on individual patients, whereas others focus on the broad needs of the entire population a system serves.

In nearly every region of the country, the move toward clinical integration is changing the roles and responsibilities of health care professionals and the way they practice. RNs are becoming increasingly important in the delivery and management of care within integrated systems, because nursing traditionally has emphasized nurturing, generative, and holistic practices (American Nurses Association, 1981). Understanding and identifying the factors of successful clinical integration is important for RNs, who will be positioned to contribute to and take on leadership roles in the design, development, and evaluation of clinical processes. However, most nursing education programs have not traditionally focused on the concepts and clinical management skills required in the integrated system environment, especially those skills required to measure and evaluate the relation between cost and quality. Nursing education must adapt to this new and changing situation.

This chapter provides a review and analysis of the changing demand for RNs as care managers. Specifically, it addresses the following:

- Industry priorities and their driving forces
- The impact of clinical integration on medical management
- Nursing's role in medical management and care management
- The imperative for revamping nursing education to provide nurses with the new skills required for care management roles
- Retooling the nursing workforce for the care management model

FACTORS AFFECTING THE DEMAND
FOR RNS AS CARE MANAGERS

As first noted in Chapter One, the health care industry has responded to demand for cost containment and quality improvement by creating integrated delivery systems. Integration has been depicted as a philosophy that unites the mission and goals of health care organizations with services and providers, particularly the health professions (Lewicki, Miller, Whitman, and Coulter, 1995). Although integrated delivery systems are defined in a variety of ways, they may generally be thought of as organizations that, through ownership or contractual arrangements, provide a full spectrum of health care services and often also include health insurance functions. To achieve coordination, the delivery system is required to deliver care and manage illness in a comprehensive fashion, with an emphasis on physical, social, psychological, and spiritual health.

Ultimately, the overarching goal of integrated delivery systems is the integration of a continuum of clinical services, which, according to experts, increases system performance. Successful clinical integration is often measured by using indicators of failed integration such as duplicate tests and procedures, medication errors, decreased patient satisfaction, and so forth. Experts debate the relationships among indicators of lack of clinical integration, but three factors consistently emerge as critical success: physician leadership, efficient and timely information systems, and alignment of system incentives.

As managed care organizations have evolved, they have further defined clinical integration in the manner depicted in Table 10.1. The table illustrates the dramatic contrast between fee-for-service and managed care environments. Whereas dis-integration was the norm in the former system, integration is fundamental to the latter.

In addition, insurers and providers have sought to identify their competitive advantage in the form of core competencies (that is, a critical set of skills, knowledge, abilities, traits, and motivations that will be distinguishable and competitive in the marketplace) that address issues of cost containment, efficiency, and qual-

Table 10.1. Evolution of Clinical Integration.

From	To
1. Managing inpatient care	1. Managing care across the system, regardless of site
2. Using prospective/retrospective cost control mechanism	2. Relying on real-time patient management systems
3. Single, clinician care management	3. Multidisciplinary team care management
4. Disintegrated system	4. Clinical congruence

ity. Recent research (Strategic Consulting Services, 1995) has identified six core managed care competencies: managing population health (medical management), bearing financial risk, building and maintaining partnerships, coordinating administrative functions, establishing and managing new and distinct cultures, and building powerful information linkages or infrastructure.

Population Health Management

The cornerstone and most challenging of these competencies is often the development of superior population health management, which in its broadest sense requires accountability and management of the health of an entire community, regardless of system membership or insurance status. Population health management requires managing not only medical care but also health promotion and disease prevention. To date, very few delivery systems or managed care entities have stepped up to the challenge of truly managing, or integrating, all factors that affect the health of an entire population (Strategic Consulting Services, 1995). However, many are implementing strategies for managing medical services.

Effective Medical Management and Clinical Integration

In this era of measurement of performance and value, the demand for results is increasingly paramount. Integrated systems, provider groups, and managed care organizations must design effective medical management programs that accomplish the goals of clinical integration and provide tangible evidence of effectiveness. Thus, the greatest challenge is to link medical management program(s) to the organization's bottom line. Those who support medical management contend that it is the most essential factor in achieving long-term business goals. However, historically, CEOs and company board members have been skeptical and slow to buy in.

Managerial leaders are most receptive when medical management's cost containment features are emphasized. Medical management addresses the 87 percent of the health care dollar that is spent on the provision and purchase of medical services (physician services, hospital care, home health, ambulatory care, prescription drugs, and other ancillary services and providers). To effectively reduce health care spending, ensure financial viability, and maintain competitive positioning, health care organizations must focus on controlling these medical costs.

Medical management programs also allow health care organizations to price competitively due to efficiency gains (for example, by directing resources to appropriate levels of care and coordination). These programs also provide avenues to focus on factors other than price (for example, quality and access). This second point is critical for differentiating a company from its competitors and maintaining satisfied customers (Strategic Consulting Services, 1995).

Figure 10.2 displays major approaches to medical management, indicating the frequency with which they are utilized by integrated delivery systems. Leading integrated delivery systems tend to rely most frequently on practice guidelines or clinical pathways in their current developmental efforts (Strategic Consulting Services, 1995). These guidelines are then used in a variety of ways, most frequently as a foundation for care management, disease management, and outcomes management programs (*Medical Group Practice Digest*, 1995).

Effective medical management and case management programs usually target one or more of the small number of diseases responsible for the majority of medical costs for the population managed by an integrated delivery system. Ac-

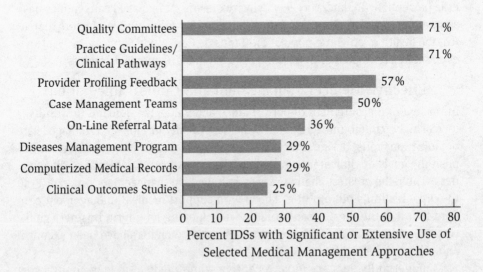

Figure 10.2. Medical Management Approaches.

Source: Strategic Consulting Services, 1995

cording to Strategic Consulting Services (1995), the most expensive medical services in the United States involve treatment of cardiovascular diseases, childbirth complications, low back pain, breast cancer, asthma, and diabetes complications.

Evidence of the effectiveness of these programs is emerging. Those with tangible, published results include case management, disease management, traditional utilization management, demand management, and selected wellness and prevention programs (Strategic Consulting Services, 1995). For example, the results of a recent Health Insurance Association of America survey indicate that insurance carriers who had invested in disability and medical rehabilitation case management programs had a thirty-to-one savings on their investment, amounting to over $50 million between 1991 and 1993. There are many other examples of such savings (Schwartz, 1996, p. 6). Moreover, research has found that the degree to which integrated systems implement strong medical management approaches indicates the systems' relative potential for enhancing value in clinical care delivery.

Nursing's Role in Medical Management

Medical management is an increasingly critical element of health services administrators' efforts to plan, organize, coordinate, finance, evaluate, and deliver care because medical management directly addresses the cost and quality of services delivered. The increased emphasis on medical management represents a great opportunity for RNs, but unfortunately one for which many of them are ill prepared.

Shortell, Gillies, and Anderson (1994) predict that within the next five to ten years nursing will likely join the dominant coalition in health services management, which for the past thirty years consisted of governing board, management, and medical staff. Shortell believes that as a professional group RNs play critical roles throughout the health care delivery system because they are typically the primary resource coordinators who are most closely linked to the critical financial and clinical data.

Nursing has historically been a critical component in setting goals and fulfilling objectives for patient care in hospitals (Schulz and Johnson, 1990). Through the 1960s, 1970s, and into the 1980s, nursing adapted to the increasing advances in technology, changing environments, and expanding scope of hospital services. As nursing expanded its degree of specialization, clinical nurse specialists, nurse clinicians, and nurse practitioners were recognized for their advanced clinical competencies and given leadership roles for newly established nursing teams.

With the advent of Medicare's prospective payment system in the mid-1980s, nurses became a critical resource to hospitals, which began to scrutinize utilization, cost, and medical necessity issues. Faced with similar pressures to contain costs, insurance companies began employing nurses to conduct utilization management, claims review, and medical record reviews, as well as to perform traditional case management functions (Kellogg Foundation, 1990). "Nurses' vast experience as first-line unit-level managers enables them to provide valuable consultation to health care organizations as they struggle to address cost and quality concerns" (Schulz and Johnson, 1990).

Today, managed care organizations and integrated systems are hiring RNs to perform in a variety of critical roles. These include managers of quality improvement strategies, evaluators of treatment, and developers of protocols, disease management programs, outcomes management programs, and care management programs (Strategic Consulting Services, 1995; Kellogg Foundation, 1990). Nursing's roles in integrated health systems also include conducting clinical research, involvement in developing clinical information systems, leading physicians in the development of clinical pathways, and other leadership roles. Evolution in the roles of nurses allows for technical nursing (cure and care services) to advance both within and outside the hospital setting but, most importantly, for professional nursing to take on greater decision-making, leadership, and executive functions (Schulz and Johnson, 1990). RNs also continue to expand their roles in health services administration. The scope and role of nursing has continued to grow outside the hospital setting, with RNs taking leadership roles in developing hospital-based home health and hospice services, as well as wellness centers (Kellogg Foundation, 1990).

A VHA Inc. and American Organization of Nursing Executives study reported in July 1996 that nursing executives are "at the heart" of the organizational redesign currently taking place in health care (Gelinas and Manthey, 1996). The survey of two thousand nursing executives was developed to study the evolving roles of nurse leaders. The study examined the changes taking place nationwide in the health care delivery system over the last few years. Of the nursing leaders surveyed, 80 percent have seen their roles and authority expand. In addition, 85 percent worked in hospitals that were currently in the midst of a redesign; nearly 60 percent said they made or make redesign decisions jointly with the CEO. The most dramatic growth in nurse executive responsibility has occurred in respiratory therapy, social services, and pharmacy. Nearly 30 percent of the nurse executives surveyed said that pharmacy services now report to them.

The survey also found that nurses are being asked to acquire additional clinical skills so they can work in more than one area and to assume more responsibility for managing patient care. These changes are paralleled by changes in the use of unlicensed assistive personnel. Half the nurses indicated restructuring has resulted in increased use of multiskilled, unlicensed personnel, especially in the phlebotomy, electrocardiogram administration, and respiratory therapy fields (Gelinas and Manthey, 1996).

From Case Managers to Care Managers

Two of the most important roles of nurses in emerging delivery systems are as case managers and care managers. Case management first appeared in the public health arena to provide coordination of community services, with nurses managing their work by caseloads (Lewicki, Miller, Whitman, and Coulter, 1995). Along a similar timeline, case management became a key function of health insurance companies, where nurses monitor and influence medical care provided to patients, typically those with a high-cost illness or disorder (Strategic Consulting Services, 1995).

The goals of case management, both historically and today, have focused on coordination, cost containment, quality of care, and collaboration. As case managers, nurses follow a process similar to physician decision making by assessing needs, developing diagnoses, planning interventions, implementing interventions, and evaluating outcomes. Nurse case managers essentially plan health care services and integrate them across the health care delivery continuum (Horn and Hopkins, 1994). The benefits of such programs are becoming increasingly important in today's environment.

Care management extends the functions and philosophies of case management (managing individual cases) to an entire population. Successful care management requires a team approach. Typically, care management teams include nurses, physicians, physician extenders, medical assistants, ancillary providers, nutritionists, psychotherapists, and other alternative care givers (Capko and Sage, 1995). Additionally, care management teams define their target population either by disease or by need (for example, prevention and education).

Tools typically used in care teams include clinical pathways, disease management programs, and benchmarking data and analyses. Often care management encompasses collecting and coordinating information from physicians, nurses, ancillary providers, managed care organizations, and the patients themselves (Strategic Consulting Services, 1995). Care management often cuts across a multitude of settings, from preventive care to home care, rehabilitation, and community care, creating an ideal mechanism for managing services and outcomes within integrated systems of care (Lewicki, Miller, Whitman, and Coulter, 1995).

Case management and care management are being implemented in hospitals to facilitate better management of care delivery and associated costs. Nursing is positioned and being called upon to lead care management teams and case management programs. As integrated systems evolve, further development of nurses' case and care management skills will be critical to success. Currently, advanced degrees (either master's or practitioner level) tend to be required by integrated systems where specialty service (high risk or chronic disease) populations are targeted, such as in oncology or obstetrics (Strategic Consulting Services, 1995). The roles for associate, baccalaureate, and master's prepared nurses will become more distinct as nurses in care and case management positions take on greater accountability for the delivery systems' performance.

CHANGING NURSING EDUCATION

What does the emergence of medical management mean for nursing education? There is clearly a serious need in the health services field for close examination of the cost-quality relationship as a routine part of system activities. Health professions education is not preparing health professionals to undertake these activities despite strong market demand for them.

Reexamining Core and Collateral Knowledge Areas

Health administrators and physicians are educated to examine either the cost *or* the quality dimension, respectively, rather than the relation between the two. Although cost-quality analysis should not be the exclusive domain of one profession, nursing is positioned to respond directly to the need to analyze the cost-quality relationship. The challenge is for nursing education to integrate cost and quality measurement techniques into the curriculum at all degree levels.

Advocating the inclusion of cost-quality knowledge development in the nursing educational system is not to say that health care is a commodity. Clearly, patients may be mistreated with an overemphasis on cost management. However, an informed analysis of the two variables simultaneously represents a responsible approach to meeting the public's needs in a managed care environment.

The Pew Health Professions Commission's report *Critical Challenges: Revitalizing the Health Professions for the Twenty-First Century* (1995) recommends a number of curricular reforms to better prepare health professionals for practice in the emerging system. Two recommendations are particularly relevant to expanding the scope and depth of the nursing curriculum to include cost-quality analysis.

The first recommendation: "All health professional schools must enlarge the scientific bases of their education programs to include the psychosocial behavioral sciences and population and health management sciences in an evidence based approach to the clinical work" (p. 22). Health professions education must encompass behavioral and social science research methods and the measurement techniques that can be applied in program evaluation and the analysis of the health behavior of specific populations.

The second recommendation: "The next generation of professionals must be prepared to practice in settings that are more intensively managed and integrated" (p. 22). RNs and other health professionals will be expected to apply the techniques of cost-quality analysis as members of interdisciplinary teams.

These teams will analyze data from integrated management and clinical information systems, develop appropriate responses, and then analyze the data again to determine whether outcome targets have been met. A sound understanding of this context is as critical to effective care management as knowledge of cost-quality analysis techniques.

Process Identification and Quality Management. Much of this interdisciplinary activity involves process identification. Process identification is based on the simple notion that all activities in the health services system can be conceived of as steps in a process of converting inputs to outputs (James, 1989). The documentation and specification of processes in health care and medical management are largely team activities. In both health services and medical management the first step in knowledge improvement is documentation and specification of measurable processes that can be controlled and managed. Process identification emphasizes control of variation and can be implemented successfully only as a recurring set of continuous efforts toward quality improvement. Quality improvement is a rapidly developing area in the health services field. This approach is not new, but typically it is underemphasized in most traditional health professions educational programs.

The techniques and functions that support process identification and quality improvement involve assessment, project management, measurement, benchmarking, and strategic analysis. The many tools of process identification and quality management include flowcharting, cause-effect diagramming, cost-benefit analysis, and relationship charting. Preparation in statistical processes and quality control analysis has a special meaning and importance in applications to health services.

Medical management is rapidly becoming a more precise knowledge area within the broader framework of health services administration. It requires knowing more about service program objectives and acquiring the tools and language for program evaluation. Medical management and associated process identification and quality improvement techniques should be a component of core knowledge in the preparation of nurses, at least at the advanced practice level.

Typically, nursing administration curriculum is offered as a graduate-level elective taught exclusively by nursing school faculty. This approach is no longer adequate. It is simply not enough to know on an elective basis a little about the administrative principles within the narrow field of nursing services. Nurses and nursing education can and should contribute more directly to an improved accounting of the quality of care and quality of the overall system.

Professional Education: Integrating Theory and Practice. The implications of these recommendations for nursing education merit specific discussion within the broader context of professional education. A professionally oriented academic program is considered strong to the degree that it effectively integrates theory and practice. The tasks of an academic program are teaching, professional service, and research. These academic tasks contribute to the identity, stability, and ultimately to the legitimization of the profession. If educators do not perform these academic tasks well the professional knowledge base and its legitimization are at stake (Abbott, 1991).

At present, academic nursing does not contribute significantly to the scope and depth of the knowledge relating to the cost-quality complexities involved in the direct provision of nursing care. Cost-quality analysis is a neglected area in the educational development of the professional nurse and too often neglected as well in the academic interests and research capabilities of nursing faculty. These are unmet responsibilities that, if addressed in nursing education curricula, could significantly improve the performance of practicing nurse professionals.

Scope and Depth of Academic Content: The Integrated Technology Curriculum. A curriculum may be defined simply as a series of structured learning sequences. That being the case, in nursing it may be instructive to think in terms of the descriptive scope of curriculum content that cuts horizontally across the disciplines such as the social and behavioral sciences while depth constitutes a vertical axis with advanced clinical study in particular specialties as its apex. One expects to find more descriptive content at the beginning levels of professional education. A curriculum builds by adding analytic depth as generic concepts are applied to phenomena within the domain of professional interest and responsibility. Nursing education must address both the scope and the depth of cost-quality phenomena. The traditional nursing curriculum not only lacks sufficient content in cost-quality analysis but also fails to progress from descriptive to more advanced and abstract analysis.

One way to examine this issue conceptually across all levels of nursing education is presented in the Integrated Technology curriculum, as illustrated in Figure 10.3. This model illustrates the academic context for nursing education. The model begins with the core knowledge areas of nursing theory and practice. Knowledge improvement analysis and tools and research methods should be added to the core knowledge areas. The collateral areas in this new model would be in epidemiology and biostatistics, medical management, and health services administration. The intended emphasis on the scope and depth of the core and collateral areas in advanced practice and graduate nursing makes the model important.

Direct patient care is the traditional clinical focus of nursing education and will not be elaborated on here. This focus extends up through advanced practice nursing. This academic content remains at the distinctive center of the nursing profession. However, at all levels nursing curricula should encompass more attention to the knowledge improvement techniques and tools, which are necessary

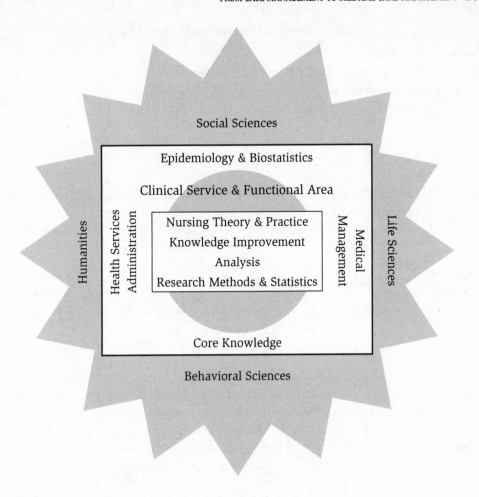

Figure 10.3. Integrated Technology Curriculum Model for Nursing.
Source: Greene, 1996

to understand the cost-quality relationship. These techniques and tools are listed in Table 10.2.

Better preparation in statistics and other research methods is especially critical. Managed care systems are much more data and information driven than the earlier institutional-based system. The nurse in the managed care environment needs an objective understanding of the content and flow of clinical and administrative work activity. Working within a context of practice guidelines, clinical pathways, and evidence-based systems requires an understanding of objective data collection and analysis. Basic concepts of validity, reliability, and so forth separate research-based standards from the criteria required to form consensus judgments. Nurse professionals need to understand and apply these concepts.

Table 10.2. Knowledge Improvement Techniques and Tools.

- KI Techniques
  Quality Improvement
  Projects and Teams
  Models for Improvement
  Tools for Process
    Description
    Flowcharts
    Cause-effect diagrams
  Models for Process Design
    Clinical paths
  Models for Strategic Planning
  Customer Needs Analysis
    Dimensions of quality
    Focus groups and surveys

- KI Tools
  For Data Collection
  Data Analysis
  Process Stability
    Control Charts
  For Collaborative Work
    Composite techniques

- Measurement Techniques
  Clinical Outcomes
  Customer Perceptions of Quality
  Internal Process
  Performance
  Financial Performance
  Benchmarking

Source: Adapted from Plsek, 1995

Basic research methods also can help the nurse professional describe and explain variation in practice. For example, understanding and controlling professional practice patterns is becoming increasingly important for health professionals of different types. Understanding the processes behind variation in practice patterns is one of the primary results of knowledge improvement analysis.

The Current Misalignment of Nursing Education

In the judgment of the authors of this chapter, nursing education at present does not effectively integrate knowledge improvement techniques and tools. This is the case across all of the degree areas and includes both the collateral and core areas recommended in the Integrated Technology model. The current levels of nursing education differentiate content based on clinical service knowledge areas (such as oncology or pediatrics) and functional areas such as nursing administration. This separation seems to diminish the development of analytic content in both the core curriculum and the collateral areas.

Nursing education curricula must be modified to place greater emphasis on analytic tools used to analyze cost-quality relationships. Understanding data collection and evaluative analysis is important at all levels of nursing education, although familiarity with research results or actually participating in research is probably not important below the baccalaureate or professional nurse level. Knowledge of the philosophy of science and the accumulation of scientific evidence also is obviously very important to comprehension of the evolution of practice guidelines as well as the establishment of evidence-based health outcomes. In addition, nurses need to know how the concepts and tools of program evaluation can be applied to process identification and quality management.

ANA Research Standards for Each Level of Nursing Education

Currently, the standards for education in research reflect the guidelines established by the American Nurses Association (ANA) Commission on Nursing Research in 1981. The commission developed standards for nursing education in research at four levels: associate, baccalaureate's, master's, and doctoral (American Nurses Association, 1981). These standards emphasize progression from consumer to scholar as an individual completes further education in nursing. The ANA commission recommended that associate and baccalaureate education focus on developing skills for consuming research, with master's and doctoral students obtaining the additional skills required to conduct research and develop theory. The standards suggest that nursing research should be primarily concerned with clinical nursing practice. However, the standards do not enumerate specific research concepts and techniques that students should acquire at each level of nursing education.

Although the ANA commission's guidelines do point to important areas of research training, the authors of this chapter think that research in nursing education should focus more on evaluative research concept skills that could be directly applied to knowledge development in the area of quality improvement and management in health services organizations. Specifically, research training should emphasize understanding of scientific methods of collecting and analyzing data in relation to practice. At the higher levels of nursing education, it should also stress integrating outside disciplinary approaches with nursing research.

In addition, the authors recommend a reevaluation of faculty competencies and the academic content of the nursing education curriculum. Nursing faculty and their academic programs need to be much more fully integrated into the broader academic community. The academic knowledge bases of all health professions are becoming increasingly interdisciplinary and cannot be advanced within the narrow limits of a professional knowledge perspective. Further, innovation in nursing education should encompass redesigning and cutting back on existing programs rather than simply adding new ones.

Matching Content with Education Level in Nursing

To ensure that RNs have the analytical tools they will need to thrive in the emerging health services environment, the authors recommend the following changes at each level of nursing education.

Associate. Associate programs should focus on professional knowledge. The descriptive aspects of nursing theory and clinical practice are best acquired and delivered at this level. Because the content is descriptive the knowledge is time bound. However, the wisdom that can accumulate through years of clinical observation should not be underestimated. The challenge is to provide a broad disciplinary conceptual base to permit valid clinical classifications for specific services and patient settings. Good clinical faculty and service settings are needed. The effective coordination of strong clinical experiences is important, yet takes nursing faculty away from the kinds of scholarly activities that are rewarded in university settings. For this reason, in associate-level programs these experiences might be better provided in new partnerships with health service systems. These systems certainly do not need to be academic health centers. In fact, educational needs may be better served in primary care settings.

Bachelor. It would seem that at this professional nurse level, the collateral and core content should be much more thoroughly examined than at present. This is where the opportunity exists to reexamine the entire four-year model to strike a better balance among the areas emphasized in the Integrated Technology model. The quality and legitimacy of academic knowledge in nursing can be strengthened if it is reconfigured in ways that build on the disciplinary scope and depth that exists on the campuses of research universities. Much experimental and demonstration work probably can be done in the health science centers of these universities, due to the availability of clinical sites and pressure to lower clinical services costs without jeopardizing quality. At the same time, new clinical partnerships are needed outside academic health centers to provide strong clinical education in primary and ambulatory care.

Advanced Practice. Understandably, associate and bachelor's degree programs are bound by college and university general education requirements and academic policies in general. Graduate and certificate programs are much less constrained. This is where the Integrated Technology model can pay off if the core and collateral areas are packaged not only in traditional degree programs, but also in certificate and nontraditional and executive program offerings.

The distinction drawn between a clinical service specialty and a functional area such as nursing administration should be reconsidered. If the core and collateral areas indicated in the Integrated Technology model can be developed, the nurse will be able to play a greater role than that of either a nursing administrator or a clinical specialist. Knowledge improvement capabilities can both contribute to the scientific base of the clinical specialist's performance and enhance the expertise of the nurse administrator.

Doctoral. The ability of nurses to gain disciplinary depth in teaching and research is an important step in the development of academic knowledge in nursing. The importance of the disciplinary method in academic programming deserves reemphasis. As the approach moves from the descriptive to the analytic and so should the rigor of nursing education. Knowledge development in the area of quality improvement and medical management content should be strongly emphasized in doctoral education programs, because doing so will strengthen the scientific base and provide analytic rigor to the course of study for both the faculty and students. The ultimate result will be a wider and deeper academic knowledge base, which in turn helps both the practice and the academic communities in which professionals serve.

Issues Surrounding Retraining of the Existing Nursing Workforce

Given the changes occurring in the health care system, many nurses will need additional education and training. A short-term solution to this problem could be the education of professional nurses in critical skill components such as cost-benefit analysis, information systems, population health management, and continuous quality improvement. Additional education in these areas, which are not likely to be a part of any RN's academic preparation, would probably contribute directly to enhanced job performance. The scope, depth, and rigor of this skill development could be adapted for different nursing degree levels and positions and levels of education.

CONCLUSION

Policymakers, analysts, and participants in the health service system agree on the priority of improving the cost-effectiveness of health care services. Because nurses are patient oriented and have a wealth of experience in direct patient care, they are in a unique position to contribute to and lead analysis of both the cost and quality dimensions of health services. Nurses' effectiveness in cost-quality analysis will be determined by both their practical experience and professional education.

Nursing has already helped direct and integrate provider teams to best serve the patient. Nurses have the opportunity to lead the health professions to a higher level of academic integration, now that teams of providers and organizations must listen to consumers and be accountable for their professional performance. As professional domains continue to be reexamined in the light of the restructuring generated by the forces of managed-care, higher levels of academic achievement and professional responsibility will be required. This will entail taking some risk by opening up the profession, collaborating in academic circles, and cutting across professional boundaries. Moreover, this will mean viewing the emerging health care environment as an opportunity to expand nurses' roles rather than as a threat to the profession.

References

Abbott, A. *The Systems of Professions.* Chicago: University of Chicago Press, 1991.

American Nurses Association. *Guidelines for the Investigative Functions of Nurses.* Kansas City, Mo.: American Nurses Association, 1981.

Capko, J., and Sage, M. J. "Care Teams: A Practical Approach to Managed Care." *American Medical News,* 1995, *38*(44), 23.

Gelinas, L. S., and Manthey, M. *The Impact of Organizational Redesign on Nurse Executive Leadership,* Part II. Irving, Tex.: VHA, 1996.

Greene, B. R. "Trends, Issues, and Models in Health Services and Health Policy Programs in Business School Settings." In P. Leatt and B. R. Greene (eds.), "Accreditation in the Health Professions," *Journal of Health Administration Education,* Winter 1996.

Horn, S., and Hopkins, D. S. "Clinical Practice Improvement: A New Technology for Developing Cost-Effective Quality." In *Health Care,* Vol. 1. New York: Faulkner & Gray, 1994.

James, B. C. *Quality Management for Health Care Delivery—Quality Measurement and Management Project.* Chicago: Hospital Research and Educational Trust, 1989.

Kellogg Foundation. *Nursing's Vital Signs—Shaping the Profession for the 1990s.* Battle Creek, Mich.: W. K. Kellogg Foundation, 1990.

Lewicki, L. J., Miller, C. M., Whitman, G. R., and Coulter, S. J. "Nursing Case Management: Coordinating a Seamless Continuum of Care." In *Integrated Health Care Delivery Systems: A Guide to Successful Strategies for Hospital and Physician.* Washington, D.C.: Thompson, July 1995.

Medical Group Practice Digest. Kansas City, Mo.: Hoechst Marion Roussel, 1995.

Pew Health Professions Commission. *Critical Challenges: Revitalizing the Health Professions for the Twenty-First Century.* San Francisco: UCSF Center for the Health Professions, 1995.

Plsek, P. E. "Techniques for Managing Quality." *Hospital and Health Services Administration,* Spring 1995.

Schulz, R., and Johnson, A. *Management of Hospitals and Health Services: Strategic Issues and Performance.* (3rd ed.) St. Louis, Mo.: Mosby, 1990.

Schwartz, M. P. "Case Management Programs Show Solid Returns." *National Underwriter Property & Casualty-Risk Benefits Management,* 1996, *3,* 6.

Shortell, S. M., Gillies, R. R., and Anderson, D. A. "The New World of Managed Care: Creating Organized Delivery Systems. *Health Affairs,* Winter 1994, pp. 46–63.

Strategic Consulting Services. *Database.* Chicago: Strategic Consulting Services, 1995.

PART FOUR

RECOMMENDATIONS FOR NURSING EDUCATION AND PRACTICE

CHAPTER ELEVEN

Nursing in the Next Century

Edward O'Neil

O'Neil closes the book by returning to the assumptions about the future environment RNs will practice in, which are first delineated in his introductory chapter and echoed throughout the book. He predicts that market forces will continue to drive the transformation of service delivery over the next five years. Although there will be some variation across regions as to when the changes will come about, most nurses will increasingly find themselves responding to issues of cost, patient satisfaction, and quality. Health care organizations will be more experimental, which will serve the interest of nurses. O'Neil presents seven broad strategic recommendations for actions, drawn from the more specific findings and recommendations presented in other chapters, that will be key to assuring nursing success in the future. The recommendations include a call for an integrated nursing practice and education continuum, and renewed focus on traditional core competencies of population-based health management and psychosocial interventions. There is also a call for strengthening research in order to demonstrate the efficacy of nursing intervention, building new partnerships, and investing in leadership development.

The chapters of this book paint dramatically variable pictures of the future of nursing practice and education. One is drawn to employ that favorite opening of high school yearbook editors, "it was the best of times, it was the worst of times." As the health care system continues its process of reinvention, all health professionals face both great opportunities and daunting threats from the changes that abound. Labor costs account for 70–80 percent of total health care expenditures. Any effort to change health care will affect the roles, requirements, and working environment of all health care workers.

As health care delivery organizations consolidate and restructure themselves, this new environment will present different career pathways for nursing professionals. At the same time it may also reduce the number of nurses needed in hospitals and other traditional settings. This may create a situation where some nurses with advanced training and skills are widely sought after, while others with entry-level training and experience find it difficult to gain employment. New candidates, such as the multiskilled allied health care worker, may be utilized to perform those tasks traditionally carried out by nurses. As systems strive for efficiency, they will look for every opportunity to substitute unlicensed assistive personnel for licensed professionals for tasks that do not require professional education and licensure.

Nurses' roles and demand for their services also will be shaped by broader demographic, socioeconomic, and scientific trends. As the nation becomes more ethnically diverse, nursing will also need to create opportunities to ensure that the profession represents the nation's population. Although the demographic bulge of the baby boom has yet to reach retirement age, it looms as a reminder that the nation is aging and will increasingly demand health services geared to an older population. The Human Genome project and other biomedical research efforts will continue to yield discoveries that will dramatically alter the prevention, diagnosis, and treatment of illness. Finally, information and communications technologies present enormous opportunities for changing the location, pattern, and structure of clinical practice. Nurses will find themselves in the midst of these and other transitions as well.

Along with growing demands for primary care providers will come new recognition of the availability and skills of nurse practitioners. They will increasingly be called upon to carry out many of the duties and tasks that have been the prerogative of physicians. This will represent an opportunity to make systems of care more affordable and perhaps more responsive to patient care needs and satisfaction, but it may also lead to conflict with physicians over scopes of practice.

As nurses are called upon to perform these new roles, there will be corresponding demands for education to provide newly minted nurses with skills to match these challenges and to retrain nurses who must incorporate these new skills into their professional practice. The opportunities are great, but so are the potential downfalls. If nursing is to flourish in the next century, nursing leaders at all levels must fully understand the nature of the transformation and make appropriate adjustments to educational programs, professional policies, and public laws governing the practice of nursing.

Forecasting changes in today's health care system might be likened to using chaos theory to explain the weather. The general patterns and trends are known, but they are being enacted over a very large-scale environment with tens of thousands of microchanges occurring daily. Collectively these microchanges add up to produce a pattern of weather that varies considerably from area to area and from season to season, yet has a definable and knowable trend. At the same time, it is impossible to predict with exactness what the weather will be tomorrow in any particular location.

Regardless of the difficulty, we should try to assemble what the chapters of this book tell us about the changing health care reality, the current status of nursing, and the likely pathways that will face the profession in the future. The authors' insights and impressions about the changing nature of nursing practice address the organization of care and service, the settings in which care is provided, and the way it has been and will be financed. Some of the perspectives offered here completely parallel one another; others are contradictory. Such is the difficulty in trying to predict the future of the rapidly changing and highly variable health care landscape.

ASSUMPTIONS ABOUT THE FUTURE

The assumptions that follow interrelate and are listed in no particular rank of importance. However, they do follow a certain logic of building on the previous assumption. These assumptions will be followed by seven recommendations for action that are structured around the themes of professional education, professional practice, the health care system, and public policy.

1. *Market and political dynamics will continue to be the dominant forces realigning the system of health care in the United States.* Professional, policy, and community forces will continue to play a role in health care, but will serve to mediate the impact of the market and politics rather than dominate the organization and financing of health care. There will be an expansion of efforts at the state and national level to promulgate a regulatory environment in which the health care market can be both efficient and responsive to public needs.

2. *Most of the health care system will make the transformation to the next generation of service delivery over the next five years.* Even those locations that seem well advanced will continue to evolve new ways to organize the delivery of care. Although this seems to be a rather rapid change for a system that has taken fifty years to develop, in reality these developments build on substantial changes that have already occurred in many parts of the country. Such changes have accelerated as market forces have come to dominate health care.

3. *Specific changes in health care will vary considerably across time, geography, and institutional setting, with urban and suburban settings being the most attractive markets for change.* Today, some areas of the country remain untouched by this revolution. However, as the market in health care becomes more voracious it will undoubtedly arrive in areas where traditional modes of organization and financing are most entrenched. The second generation of movement to managed systems will likely go faster because its leaders can draw upon lessons learned in regions where such systems already dominate. In addition, the consolidation of capital in health care is concentrating resources in the hands of entrepreneurs eager to expand market share.

4. *The emerging market will value services furnished by nurses and others as they make a contribution to three outcomes: controlling costs, enhancing consumer satisfaction, and improving the quality of outcomes.* The relative importance of these factors will vary from market to market, but collectively they will remain

paramount. Most markets are now focusing on cost and patient satisfaction. However, as excess capacity is extracted from the system, the capacity to add value by improving the outcomes with alternative approaches to delivery will become increasingly important. The most forward-thinking health care organizations are already embarking on a health improvement agenda that promises to yield long-term changes in the ways costs are controlled and quality is improved. In any given market, health care organizations will have two kinds of consumers: individuals and large corporate purchasers. These two groups will bring different values and expectations to their encounters with the health care system.

5. *The market will continue to develop and use managed systems of care as the principle mechanisms for making health care more responsive to cost, consumer satisfaction, and health outcomes.* Two major types of managed care plans are emerging in this marketplace. In recent years, there has been considerable growth in those parts of the health care system that represent more open, networked, or virtual systems of care. In these arrangements, managed care companies contract for services with physician groups, hospital systems, home nursing agencies, and other health care providers. The system is a virtual one in that the managed care or insurance company joins those inputs that meet their needs for cost control, consumer satisfaction, and overall quality. The alternative to such an approach is vertical integration, in which a single entity that owns or controls all inputs, such as a staff-model HMO or a provider-owned delivery system, provides a full spectrum of management, professional, and institutional services. Each approach has its strengths and weaknesses. Virtually integrated systems are more flexible, whereas vertically integrated systems are better positioned to standardize clinical and organizational processes. It seems likely that these two approaches will be balanced in the future. Regardless of which strategy is pursued, the health care system will be marked by increased consolidation of providers, both within service groups and across geography.

6. *As systems gain more control over the various inputs necessary to produce health care and as consolidation of health care providers yields fewer options for purchasers (individual or corporate), health care delivery systems will more aggressively experiment with alternative ways to deliver services.* The market values just described will continue to drive systems' goals, but systems will have more freedom to develop innovative and creative alternatives for achieving these goals. As such innovations evolve, there will be both more opportunity for new entities to enter the market and fewer enfranchised prerogatives for institutions and professionals within the system. This new competitive environment will do more to alter the fundamental relationships of these institutions and professionals than anything else in this century.

7. *The changes that are coming about are made possible in large measure by the information and communications technologies that will become available*

over the next decade. Technology is not driving change in health care but rather is a critical tool for implementing change. Information has been at the root of what has kept health care segmented and specialized; the emergent technology may foster its reintegration. The availability of this technology will facilitate system change in several important ways. First, advances in data collection, storage, analysis, and distribution will permit providers to access both individual and population health data during clinical encounters. Second, powerful tools for linking and quickly analyzing large data sets will facilitate more systematic and intensive management from a population perspective than was possible in the past. Finally, the technology will lead to better access to information by consumers, enabling them to assume increasing levels of responsibility for their own health and care.

8. *Intervention by federal and state government policies and professional associations will not stop the transformation of the health care system.* For-profit institutions may not dominate the health care industry, but they do set and will continue to set the standards for efficiency and consumer responsiveness. To remain competitive, community-based and nonprofit institutions will find it necessary to meet the standards set by the for-profits. The best that policymakers can strive for is the creation of a regulatory envelope that protects individuals, encourages the market to work efficiently, and ensures that population approaches to health care are valued and used. Perhaps the best professional associations can do is to help their members understand the emerging system. They will also be useful as they assist members in accommodating to the requirements of this new order and seizing the opportunities it presents. The nursing profession must not succumb to the temptation to resist these inevitable changes in health care. Instead it should actively position itself to play a leadership role in the transformation in order to better serve the public.

SEVEN STRATEGIES TO POSITION NURSING FOR THE NEXT CENTURY

This dynamic environment presents both peril and opportunity for all professions. Some appear better positioned to take advantage of the changes than others. The professions themselves and the associations that serve them can strengthen their position by anticipating as best they can the changing environment and moving their members to respond constructively. Actions professional associations should take include assessing the profession's current roles, developing scenarios for the future, and retooling professional practice and education to prepare professionals for enhanced roles. Some professional associations are already engaged in this work, but much more remains to be done.

The movement by the professional pharmacy community over the past decade toward the preparation of clinical pharmacists offers one example of a constructive response by a profession to changes in the environment. During the early 1980s, it became increasingly obvious that the traditional dispensing function of pharmacists would disappear with growing cost consciousness, changes in technology, and potential substitution of other workers. As a result, the professional pharmacy community began asking where on the continuum of care pharmacists added value to patients and systems of service. The profession's leaders broadened the definition of their services beyond the delivery of a pharmaceutical product to include such responsibilities as working with other clinicians to promote effective use of pharmaceuticals, educating patients about their medications, and the direct delivery of services as part of a team of providers when complex patient care needs required a more active role for the pharmacist.

This broadened role for the pharmacist necessitated a revamped and expanded educational program. The proposal met with considerable resistance within the profession and from other interests, such as chain drug stores. The leadership persevered with the reform agenda and today all academic programs have committed to moving to a Pharm.D. degree, with its focus on pharmaceutical care, by early in the next century.

This transition was successful for several reasons that are important to discuss here. First, the movement was born out of a frank and realistic assessment of the environment. Pharmacists did not deny or attempt to halt the dramatic changes in the health care environment. Leadership was also key to the change. Without the commitment of a sizable part of the profession's leaders to push this agenda, it would have met an early and untimely doom. The third and perhaps most critical element of their success was not expecting to receive full endorsement of their ideas from all involved. Rather, the relatively small leadership cadre built a movement that changed much of the expectations of the profession.

By adapting to change rather than resisting it, pharmacy has positioned itself to play a leadership role in the emerging managed care systems. What comparable steps should the nursing community take to improve its position in the coming transition? Historically, nursing has been driven by the vagaries of the health care market. Indeed, nursing education has its roots in turn-of-the-century hospitals' efforts to meet growing demands for services. This focus on immediate needs has yielded a capacity for flexibility unequaled among health care providers, but it has also inhibited nursing's ability to institute long-term changes. Long ago, nursing recognized the need to rationalize the entry into practice and the relationship between levels of training and work. Yet the profession is still burdened with three entry points to practice and general confusion regarding the different roles played by nurses with various levels of education.

Seven distinct ideas emerge as essential for the renewal of nursing practice and education. They represent strategic directions for nursing. As such, they present a broad outline rather than a detailed blueprint for action. They are intended to form a vision within which nursing leaders can implement specific changes at national, state, and local levels.

Create an integrated continuum for nursing practice.

As the nation's largest health profession, nursing will find the impact of changes in the health care system magnified. The profession has prided itself on being a single profession regardless of level of preparation or experience. One of the great strengths of nursing is the common clinical core experience that is a part of all levels of nursing education. Nursing's orientation toward the management of care will increasingly be one of the most-needed elements in the new system. Such an orientation has been possible only because basic nursing education is not specialized.

However, the new system will create more and more opportunities for health professionals who have richer arrays of skills and competencies. Many opportunities in the emerging health care system will demand differentiation, if not outright specialization. Some nurses continue to cleave to the concept that a nurse is a nurse, in part because of their shared introductory clinical experience. This idea must be jettisoned because it no longer serves the patient, the public, the health care institution, or the profession.

Nursing as a profession must begin to work toward a shared articulation of the competencies and likely practice settings for nurses along a continuum of professional practice. What are the core competencies that distinguish an associate from a baccalaureate-trained RN? Have these core competencies been adjusted to meet the changing needs of the health care system and should they be adjusted further if there is movement to create a continuum of practice as indicated here? How does an experienced RN add value differently from that of a newly minted nurse? What are the changes in practice settings and independence of practice that should occur as the nurse moves along an educational and practice continuum? Addressing these matters is hard work and emotionally debilitating for many in the profession, but it is essential to position the profession to add value to the new care delivery systems that will exist in the next century.

The nursing community should identify a continuum for nursing practice. However, if the profession fails to act the health system will impose its own rationalization to meet its changing care delivery needs. In fact, such divisions are already made informally in many settings. Clearly, the common core of clinical skills should be the base upon which all nursing professional roles are built. This core may be represented in the curriculum at the associate degree level and should represent preparation into entry-level positions in the most supervised environments.

The nurse emerging from this entry-level position will have many different options to pursue. Some have always been a part of nursing and others are more relevant to the new systems of care. Of particular importance are the roles of the nurse as clinical team leader, mid-level system manager of patients and populations, and deliverer and coordinator of outreach services. It would seem that these roles require different levels and kinds of experience that all build on the clinical core. These practice domains might appropriately be met by the added value of baccalaureate training, but should also be carried out in part by individuals with training in the core disciplines who have demonstrated competence in these areas in a formal manner.

Finally, there are more advanced roles for nurses in clinical and leadership positions. Advance practice nurses are being called upon to carry out more extensive roles in care delivery systems. As these systems create more opportunity for nursing clinical practice, these roles will undoubtedly expand in both inpatient and ambulatory settings. The system also needs nurses with advanced management and systems training in executive leadership roles. Professionally prepared nurses in these positions will be extremely valuable as they build upon their core clinical education and experience and apply it to redesign the delivery of health services.

These clinical service pathways should be structured in such a way as to accommodate lifelong learning of nurses. Convenient exit and reentry points for further training, from entry level through doctoral level study, should facilitate the movement of the nurse along the continuum of nursing practice. This restructuring of nursing is necessary for the profession to take full advantage of the opportunities that the changing health care system presents. Moreover, the profession has the responsibility to respond to these challenges.

Create a continuum of education that supports the practice continuum.

An individual might enter a particular level of nursing practice directly by extending the period of initial training or by returning for more advanced training as opportunity and personal decisions mandate. Today, nursing may have the best internal career ladder among the health professions. But additional work must be done to identify the practice domain and core competencies at each level of nursing practice and training if nursing is to respond effectively to the demands of the emerging health care environment.

In the long run, the profession will be served best by carefully identifying the level of competency needed for effective nursing practice in each role and setting. Nursing education programs must ensure that they are offering a set of experiences that foster these competencies and that they do so in the most effective and efficient manner. In addition, RNs must see themselves as lifelong learners, seeking out opportunities to upgrade and refine their skills. As with nursing practice, the care delivery system may find that direct intervention to train the workers it needs is more efficient than trying to get the attention of educators.

Ultimately, creating parallel continuums of nursing practice and education could mean that the educational process may diverge from licensure. Such a position is often contentious and counterintuitive to the perceived interests of any profession. In fact, the movement to managed systems of care has made most health professions increasingly more defensive about professional ownership of scopes of practice. Such a step would be a bold statement by nursing. It would be an affirmation that the profession had thought carefully and broadly about the changing competencies needed for successful practice in the new health care system. It would also signal that the profession has structured these competencies in a logical developmental sequence and ensure that the educational programs sanctioned by the profession provide the most effective and efficient set of experiences to achieve these competencies. Membership in the profession would be the gold standard for a prospective employer to ensure that an individual possesses the competencies to add value to the health system.

Focus the profession on two core competencies.

The first impulse for the development of an integrated continuum of nursing practice and a complementary educational continuum will be to focus on the clinical core of nursing. This is important and necessary, but not sufficient to reposition the profession of nursing for the next century. Beyond the needed focus on core clinical skills is the identification and affirmation of core competencies that have always been a part of nursing and that integrated systems of care will increasingly demand. Two related competencies seem particularly important: population-based approaches to health and the incorporation of the psychosocial-behavioral perspective into the delivery of care.

Population-based health means moving beyond the provision of treatment services to individuals as they present acute care needs. This approach to health care requires that the individual, practice, institution, or system take as its unit of analysis the whole population. This will require nursing professionals to understand the concepts and tools of epidemiology and apply them in a variety of contexts, ranging from individual patient encounters to the management of complex systems. Such an orientation also means that nursing professionals must have the skills necessary to assess the health of a population and the capacity to develop a set of outcomes or health goals for that population. Additionally, nursing professionals must be able to determine the most effective way to allocate increasingly limited resources to achieve these goals and to lead individuals or organizations in implementing pathways for effective delivery of services.

This approach to population health and the skills associated with it are at the core of the nursing profession. They are drawn from the profession's basic orientation of care rather than cure. They also come from the profession's historical work in large institutions, public health settings, and the community. But these skills and orientations must be adapted to the new realities and demands of integrated systems of care. This will challenge nursing professionals to rethink how they approach case management, manage within institutions, provide clinical care, work with other professionals, and provide leadership for the system.

Of particular importance will be the ability to use effective analytical skills to control costs and improve quality. The intensive work of changing the patient encounter and managing it in a way to achieve lower costs and higher quality must be led by health professionals. Nurses have the opportunity to take up this challenge, but they must demonstrate that they can deliver these results. To do so, nurses will need better education in the application of analytic tools to the management of health care delivery.

In its focus on care, nursing has always incorporated a larger range of perspectives regarding the determinants and outcomes of health than those encompassed by the biomedical model. In particular, nursing has done more than other professions to incorporate the psychosocial-behavioral perspective into a full range of clinical practice competencies. This orientation shapes the ways nurses deliver care to individuals, design and manage institutions, and think about the population values within entire systems of care.

These two core competencies of serving populations and understanding care in the broad psychosocial-behavioral context will be of increasing value to the emerging care delivery systems. The nursing profession, of course, does not "own" these competencies, and other professions have their own ways of demonstrating ability in these domains. The challenge will be for nursing to strengthen nurses' competencies in these domains and demonstrate why they are uniquely positioned to apply these competencies to the delivery of health care services. For the future, nursing practice and education would benefit from pushing their understanding of these values in the context of the new systems of care. The insights derived from such a process should directly inform the educational and practice continuum described earlier.

If movement in this direction is accepted by the educational part of the profession, the temptation will be to add course work in this area to what is perceived as an already crowded curriculum. A better strategy would be to design a set of educational experiences outside the box of the existing program, aggressively tying such a development to the needs of a radically different health care delivery system.

Strengthen the professional commitment to research.

In part, professional identification means a commitment to understanding and advancing a body of knowledge. However, nursing emerged as a practice-driven profession that has assembled its theoretical and research underpinnings in order to understand the phenomena that practice has presented. Although it may have been seen as a weakness of the profession, this precise orientation has led the profession to value the competencies in population health and psychosocial-behavioral matters that are so important to the new approach to health care.

The distinctive competencies of nursing must be advanced by a much more intentional, perhaps even directed, research agenda from the profession. The emerging system of care will value those inputs that can demonstrate a positive contribution to outcomes for both the individual and the population. Individual professionals and entire professions will have to make the case for themselves based on objective, empirical measures of positive contribution to outcomes. Many of these data collection projects will take years to design and carry out. In fact, one refreshing element of the emerging system seems to be an ongoing commitment to experimentation and improvement. But this means that it may become much more important for a profession to control and advance its research agenda than to control the scope of its practice in traditional ways. In fact, one could argue that the future control of scopes of practice will be a function of research in outcomes, not the actions of legislators.

Some research in nursing is already focused on issues of outcomes and evidence-based approaches to improving the health status of patients. However, this research remains isolated within the body of nursing research. Strengthening nursing's knowledge base in outcomes research should be the central concern of the profession.

Reduce the number of nurses educated in associate degree and diploma programs.

Nursing education programs, like all parts of the health care system, expanded over the past thirty years. This expansion was in response to a growing hospital system and the need for nurses to staff these facilities. Not only has that system stopped growing, it is poised for considerable contraction by a reduction in hospital beds and closure of many hospitals. Such changes will inevitably affect the employment prospects for RNs, particularly at the entry level.

Although it is impossible to know the exact nursing skills needed in the emerging systems, it is likely that value will be placed on an efficient pathway for individuals to enter the system. The associate degree provides such an entry point, but affords only a limited basis for professional development. In addition, associate degree programs have emphasized preparation for practice in hospitals, as have the diploma programs that are already vanishing from the nursing education landscape. There simply will be fewer opportunities for RNs educated solely as generalists at the associate degree or diploma level. Adaptation to the emerging environment will require reduction in their numbers.

The baccalaureate degree may offer some additional time to training, but cannot be a substitute for advanced training or experience. Although nursing should value all pathways, it is critical that the profession develop education programs that are flexible, more integrated into the continuum of practice, and able to evolve with both the individual professional and the needs of the care delivery system. Nursing will need to be open to exploring creative alternatives for achieving these goals. The associate-to-master's-degree bridge programs already in operation should be looked to as one approach to addressing these issues.

Create strategic partnerships for nursing.

For the past five decades the U.S. health care system has built a tremendously complex system of care. One of the elements of the complexity has been the segregation of care into discrete professional domains—nursing, medicine, pharmacy—and the separation of processes associated with health into equally discrete institutions—public health, hospital, clinic, finance. What seems likely in the future is that much of what has been separated will be reconnected, particularly when the reunion produces positive system outcomes.

Because nursing is so central to most systems of care, it is in an excellent position to become essential to many of the partnerships that will emerge. Nursing should be strategic in choosing its partnerships. Choices should be made in a way that enhances the ability of the profession to contribute its core competencies in population and psychosocial health. These choices will vary over time and place, but some general alignments of interests seem to be emerging.

In health care delivery, thoroughly integrated systems are likely to make better partners than the parts of the system that still operate independently. A system is able to look across a full range of service needs and has the independence to create innovative approaches to meet those needs. The independent components of a system, such as hospitals, seem more likely to maintain their traditional biases for organization and financing of care and may not have interests that reach beyond their institutional walls. Nurses will find partnerships with such organizations difficult as the missions and strategies of professions and health care institutions move toward further integration. Without an agreement to create something new, nursing educators and hospital leadership will find themselves more often at an impasse than at a creative juncture to reengineer the health care delivery process.

The academic health center has been the leader in health professional education. But this arena has been so dominated by academic medicine that for the most part other professions have not been adequately integrated into these institutions. Moreover, academic health centers face a difficult decade as they redefine their own mission and move to new mechanisms of finance. As nurses look for partnerships for education they might look to the care delivery system or health care plan, as well as to the schools and colleges that have been nursing's traditional partners. Is it wise for the profession to look to the practice world for educational partners after having so recently left the hospital or diploma school for the academic organization? This is a legitimate concern. However, the practice and educational worlds have evolved considerably in the past fifty years, and nursing education and the emerging health care systems have complementary needs and resources.

Research in health professions has grown around the biomedical model funded essentially by the National Institutes of Health. Nursing professionals have made significant inroads into this funding source, and they should continue to develop and carry out projects in this modality. The most promising new research partnerships for nursing, however, are in those areas where their strengths in population health and psychosocial-behavioral health integrate with the interests of the emerging system and where pursuit of these interests can be combined with the clinical research work of nurses. Disease management, demand management, and population assessment are all areas that nursing has demonstrated an ability to address through research. The health care systems themselves are the most likely sources of support for future work in these areas. Nursing researchers should begin working now to develop such partnerships.

Invest in enhancing leadership.

Finally, each of these transformations in health care and nursing will come about only if leaders are present at all levels—national, state, professional, institutional—to identify the opportunities and move the profession toward them. The profession of nursing, along with all of the health professions, is confronted with a stark and unsettling reality. The organization and delivery of care is changing dramatically. Some of the changes will benefit nursing; others are undoubtedly distasteful. The ability of any organized profession to respond to these changes is limited by the traditional values and orientations of the professions and by the essential conservative nature of professional life and values. The nursing profession's dominant mode of response today is an organized, and at times unionized, effort aimed at saving jobs. Though the use of such response is probably inevitable during a time of transition, if it becomes the only response of the nursing profession, it will tend to isolate the profession from decision making about the future of the health care delivery systems in which its members work.

Leadership is the antidote to such reactions. But to be successful it must be informed, developed, and integrated. Informed means the ability to step outside the professional box and see how the world is changing. Not all that is going on in the transition of health care is pleasant, but all of it must be seen and understood for leaders to begin to know how to plan and how to act. But knowing is not enough; leaders must also develop the skills for action. Health care has been a heavily regulated industry that neither valued nor needed entrepreneurial-type action. This is no longer the case; entrepreneurship will be a critical element of nursing leadership in the emerging system. Finally, nursing leadership must be integrated across the various factions within nursing that have historically divided the profession. This division is the greatest single obstacle to nursing achieving the promise of the future that is set out in this book.

The complexity and size of the challenge of changing health care in the United States is daunting and can be defeating for some. As big as this challenge is, it is precisely its magnitude and dramatic nature that create an enormous opportunity for nurses and the nursing profession. But this does not mean nursing will be permitted to defend its turf better and resist change longer. In fact, the opportunity will be seized by those individuals and professions that are quick to see the parallels between the basic values of the new system and the values of their own profession. This book has attempted to produce some insights into those patterns of overlap.

But in the final analysis it will be the leadership of the nursing profession that makes the transformation successful or not. Just as with the pharmacy profession remaking itself, nursing has certain strengths and opportunities as well as certain weaknesses and threats. Will the leadership get caught in the old patterns of relating between nursing and other professions, or will it work constructively to create a new governance and relational basis for the profession? Will the leadership defend what is, rather than create what could be? Will the profession cover up weaknesses and places where it may come up short, or will it have the courage to ask and answer new questions?

Like all of the health professional bodies in the United States, nursing is dominated by the professional association and member governance structure. When there was no bottom line in health care these structures were adequate, because resources were not a concern and no one questioned the authority of the professions to make decisions relevant to their work. The times are and will continue to be different. Now, professional workers must prove their relevance to the mission of the emerging systems of care. They will not prove it through lawsuits and strikes, but by the concerted effort to assess what is important about health care change and to understand how they might relate and contribute to the new patterned ways of practicing. These are leadership questions and issues facing nursing leaders as the profession moves into the next century.

This could be the dawning of a new age for nursing. Achieving this promise will fundamentally depend upon the leaders of the profession from the schools to the associations to the practice settings. May they be equal to this formidable challenge.

NAME INDEX

SUBJECT INDEX

J